S
GHT
AT AGE 65

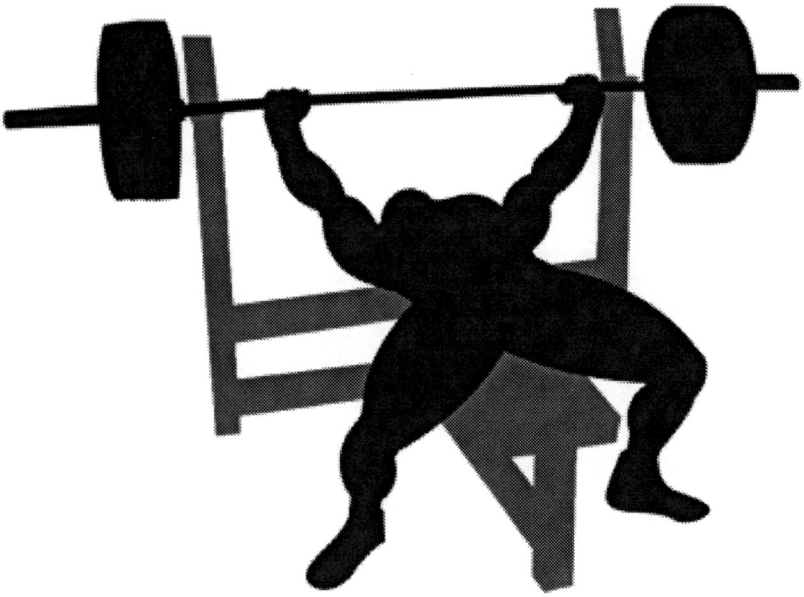

The incredible benefits of strength training that can reverse your biological age by 20 years and extend your healthy lifespan by decades

by

William Faro – the living proof

ISBN: 978-1-905006-74-8

A C.I.P reference is available from the British Library.

Printed and bound in Great Britain.

TABLE OF CONTENTS

Illustrations

INTRODUCTION

The First Dumbbell

Since leaving school I had not seen the inside of a gym until well into my late forties. I picked up my first dumbbell just after my fiftieth birthday. Prompted, I think, by an article I chanced across on the benefits of strength in old age. At the time I was reasonably fit and certainly not overweight but I was also at that stage of life when it starts to sink in that this really is the only body I've got. It is literally my only contact with reality. How long do I want to keep it working? How long do I want to retain total mobility and thus independence?

Your body is the only possession you own absolutely - outright. There may be a few spare parts available nowadays but no replacements. Castles, money, titles, lovers and sundry other seemingly indispensable possessions can be acquired, but they can be lost - they can be taken from you. Only death can steal your body. The state of your body dictates your lifestyle to a devastating extent. Without a vital body all other possessions are rendered useless. As if those were not reasons enough to look after it, I felt that chancing on that article might have been one of fate's subtle hints prompting me to investigate further.

So I started to investigate, and then to appreciate, the unbelievable number of benefits of increased strength in old age. I came across scientific studies indicating a complete slow down (and in many cases reversal) in the ageing processes by performing rational, efficient strength training that increases muscle mass and bone density. I discovered a host of other benefits ranging from lower blood pressure to loss of body fat. From reduced 'bad' cholesterol to increased 'good' cholesterol. From increased testosterone levels to improved insulin sensitivity. From a strengthened immune system to naturally increased production of human growth hormone.

The evidence was overwhelming and compelling. But could all these benefits really flow from just hoisting bits of iron into the air? There was only one way to find out for sure. I decided to be my own guinea pig.

So I started. I started with my first dumbbell at age 50 with absolutely no prior knowledge of, or interest in, bodybuilding, weight lifting or any other form of strength training. At that time I had a fairly sedentary management position in the visual arts, keeping reasonably fit through tennis, swimming and intermittent skiing. But when I picked up that first dumbbell I became inspired. I felt I was doing something that nature intended. Strength seemed to be a totally natural attribute of a healthy body. This is not surprising really when you consider that for many hundreds of thousands of years, right up to the comparatively recent start of so called civilisation in fact, strength was the most essential quality to ensure survival. So I jumped in with both feet.

At 51 I was stronger than I had been in my thirties and forties. Today, at over 65, I bench press my bodyweight with comparative ease and am stronger than I have ever been in my life. Not only stronger but also healthier in mind, body and spirit. I have not had a serious cold in years, a direct result, I believe, of a stronger immune system.

A Practical Fountain of Youth

It is now a generally accepted medical fact that the benefits of resistance training are a practical fountain of youth. A means of literally rolling back the years by altering your biological age as scientifically measured by a standard set of biomarkers of ageing - one of the many benefits of increased strength.

This book is about the 18 crucial benefits of resistance training (Part 1) that I have identified and experienced (there are doubtless many others) and exactly how to achieve them through building strength efficiently, in the shortest possible time (Part 2). Most importantly, the workouts can be incorporated into a busy lifestyle in the most practical manner. They are short and simple, with the sole objective of increasing Lean Body Mass.

My Own Guinea Pig

Part 2 covers every aspect of practical strength building in what I believe is the most efficient manner in order to achieve identical results as mine. The optimal routines I describe are the result of experimenting over the last 15 years with many different training programs. I have trained Mondays, Wednesdays and Fridays. I have trained different body parts once a week, once a fortnight and even once a month when I was investigating Static Contraction Training. I have under trained and over trained and suffered accordingly. I have experimented with all manner and combinations of, sets, supersets and repetitions. I really have been my own guinea pig. I have suffered setbacks, 'plateauing', and injury; and learnt how to completely avoid all of these conditions.

The Living Proof

I have proved that anyone at age 50 (or at any age) can take up strength training and immediately start reaping the massive benefits. I have gone on to bench press my body weight and demonstrate that further improvement is possible into my mid sixties – as I know it will also be in my mid seventies, for which I have set new higher goals. Although for obvious reasons I cannot prove that just yet my progress towards these goals will be monitored on my website www.williamfaro.com which also features many useful articles, updates and links, and which offers readers free help and support.

But I will prove it in due course – for the very good reason that my biological age is now somewhere in the mid forties, back where I was before I picked up my first dumbbell. I am now able to view the next 20 years from that perspective, rather than from that of my chronological age of over 65 and plan my future life accordingly. I have, quite simply, bought more useable time. More time to enjoy family, friends and loved ones and more time to develop a completely new career. That is exactly what I have become inspired to do.

It is never too late to start. Research on elderly subjects has shown that just 2 months of strength training can reverse 2 decades of strength and muscle loss. In one study a group of men in their sixties and seventies increased hamstring and quadriceps (thigh muscles) strength by 227% and 107% respectively. The list goes on. But it is vital ***to*** start if you want to be living in your body, rather than dying in it.

If you are still in any doubt as to whether resistance training is for you please just glance at the table of contents which lists the 18 crucial benefits of increased strength that I have identified (and there must be many more). If that is not sufficient a carrot for you I recommend jumping straight to Chapter 30 'The Downside' where you will find the alternatives.

Strength training is for everyone. Whatever your age or sex you can reap the enormous life changing benefits that flow from a stronger body. With increasing life expectancy, these benefits will become absolutely vital for every man and woman, as their 60's and 70's approach, in order to maintain total independence and dignity right into advanced old age.

Remember, I started with absolutely no knowledge or experience whatsoever at age 50. Everything in this book I have tried and tested. I really am the living proof. You can be too.

Just decide that a walking stick, let alone a Zimmer frame, will never, ever, figure in your future. Set a target to bench press your bodyweight and I will give you every possible support. With my best wishes.

William Faro

Part 1:
The Incredible Benefits of Strength Training

Chapter 1

Benefit 1: Rollback Your Biological Age by Decades and Look Years Younger

Have you ever seen an 80-year-old man with massive shoulders, 6-pack abs, bulging biceps and python arms? Probably not. At least that is what you assume. When you come across someone with this physique you naturally age him about 20 years younger than his real age - because that is how he looks. Your brain is telling you that muscle equals youth. You are assessing him on his biological, rather than on his chronological, age.

His physique looks 60, and since you only have looks to go on, you consider this to be his age. That he was born 80 years ago is quite irrelevant to his looks, health and lifestyle - and most importantly it is also quite irrelevant to his future longevity.

> Worry not about when you were born, for it is your biological age which determines when you will die

Only your chronological age can be measured by the calendar. Your true or biological age is a much more accurate guide to your future longevity. There are several well-established biomarkers of ageing that are used to give more accuracy to the assessment of physiological age.

One of the principal ones is the amount of muscle your body contains - Lean Body Mass or LBM (see Chapter 2). The more muscle you have, the younger you are biologically. Another biomarker of ageing is bone density (see Chapter 3). So what is the number one method of increasing both LBM and bone density? You probably guessed it - strength training.

Not only is muscle or Lean Body Mass one of the principal biomarkers, it is the one that is immediately apparent, which is why I have listed looking younger as the number one benefit of building strength through weight training. You have to look pretty long and hard to assess a person's cholesterol levels, or insulin sensitivity but strong defined muscles toned by weight training stand out a mile.

Biomarkers are all accurately measurable, and the results indicate a specific maturity, which is why they were chosen; hence a scientific way of measuring your biological age. As well as LBM and bone density other biomarkers include:-

- Body Fat Percentage
- Muscle Strength
- Aerobic Capacity
- Metabolism (Basal Metabolic Rate or BMR)
- Blood Pressure
- Cholesterol Levels (HDL/LDL ratios)
- Insulin Sensitivity

Most of the above are easily and cheaply measured by your doctor, pharmacist and/or physical trainer. Regardless of your chronological age the results may show, for example, that your blood pressure is that of a normal 25-year-old, your body fat percentage equivalent to that of a 32-year-old and your muscle strength that of a 28 year old etc.

The average of the results will provide a fairly accurate indication of how far you are behind or, heaven forbid, even ahead of your chronological age. The good news is that whereas you can do absolutely nothing about your chronological age every single one of the biomarkers that makes up your biological age is directly under your control. Moreover, ***every single one of them is improved by strength training.***

As your muscles grow and your level of fitness increases you will start to improve (reduce) your biological age by altering all the biomarkers of ageing. Your level of health will improve dramatically and often revert to that of a person 20 years younger. Your looks will also improve and not only due to the changes that are taking place within your body, but also due to the much increased energy and vitality which always give a strong perception of youthfulness. You will not only look younger but also actually ***be*** biologically younger.

Exactly how much younger you will look is to some extent governed by other factors such as past exposure, or over exposure, to the sun or hair loss, both of which can occur at any age and so cannot be used as scientific biomarkers of ageing. I am sure, like me, you have noticed men of 30 who are already practically bald and yet others in their 70's who still have a full head of hair. If you are bald when you start strength training I regret you will still be bald 12 months down the line. However, you will still look younger than when you started.

Ironically the older you are when you start the greater the number of years younger you will look. For example a person aged 60 will very easily be able to look 10-15 years younger after say 12 months of strength training. However, had the same person started at age 30 it is unlikely he would look much younger after the same period of training.

Regardless as to what extent your looks may improve, your biological age will almost always improve further. We are all unique and will achieve differing results. In my case, aged 65, it is generally agreed I can get away with looking 55, just some 10 years younger. However, my biological age based on the biomarkers of ageing is much closer to 45 - and that is exactly the age I feel - completely devoid of any ailment as I am (even a mild irritation I noticed in my knee at age 53 just vanished years ago). This is the real number one benefit of strength training. This is what is so exciting to me - being able to plan so many more useful decades ahead. I now plan my life from the basis that I ***am*** in my late forties.

Since many of us are slightly overweight I feel others, like me, will be as equally excited about the second benefit of strength training – the reduction in body fat.

Chapter 2

Benefit 2: Reduce Body Fat and Increase Lean Body Mass

Adding muscle, or Lean Body Mass (LBM), to your body increases your Basal Metabolic Rate which means you will naturally burn more calories and lose fat 24 hours a day. Every pound of muscle burns at least 35 calories a day just to maintain itself, and that is while it is doing absolutely nothing. Adding just 5 pounds of new muscle will burn off 15 to 20 more pounds of fat annually – assuming no alteration in your calorie intake in any way. The more muscle you have the more calories you burn even when the body is at rest – even when you are fast asleep.

The more muscle you have also increases the rate at which you burn calories during exercise. Thus two people exercising for exactly the same period of time, and at the same difficulty level, on an exercise bike, for example, will burn a different amount of calories. The one with the greater LBM will burn more calories. Building LBM is the most natural and efficient way of reducing body fat there is – bar none. Exactly how to build those muscles is covered fully in Part 2.

Here is why cutting calories alone will not and, in the long run, cannot ever work. The minute you cut calorie intake significantly (as required by most diets) your body assumes a famine has occurred and immediately looks for ways to lower your metabolism in order to conserve energy and fat. As we have already seen muscles are burning up calories just by being there. Accordingly the body will switch to burning muscle for fuel while conserving fat (which requires less than 1 calorie a day to maintain itself) – the exact opposite result of what the diet intended!

This physiological law results from thousands of millennia of shortages and famine during which the body evolved this survival technique. The body has no means of distinguishing between a genuine famine and voluntary fasting. To lose fat you have to persuade your body to burn fat as the preferred fuel, which is done best during low intensity exercise such as brisk walking, and at the same time to feed it plentifully and with the right nutrients (see Chapter 27 'Nutrition').

Your body must feel that there is plenty of food available (including the right fats) so that there is no need for it to conserve fat. Then your metabolism must be raised to burn off the fat – and that is done by increasing the proportion of LBM to body fat (i.e. building more muscle) in your overall body weight which may actually increase slightly, because muscle weighs more than fat.

The ideal formula to lose fat therefore is to increase your metabolism (by building muscle) combined with low intensity aerobic exercise such as fast walking. I have recently incorporated walking into my routine with amazing results. By walking briskly for 3 to 4 miles first thing most mornings on an empty stomach I have found that my waist has become slimmer and my muscles now appear more defined – because I am burning fat for fuel. The results are in fact so spectacular that I have ceased any other aerobic activity when in the gym, apart from warming up, so I can concentrate exclusively on building muscle when there.

Brisk walking has achieved what years of painful, joint jarring jogging failed to do. I have now discovered why. The minute you move from a low intensity exercise such as walking to a higher intensity one (jogging for example) your pulse rate increases, along with puffing and panting which is a sure sign that your bloodstream is struggling to deliver sufficient oxygen to your muscles. It is at this point that the exercise has ceased to be aerobic. It is at this point that your body will switch from using fat for fuel to using glycogen instead - so no more fat burning.

Some athletes can lope along gracefully with virtually no increase in breathing rate. For those lucky specimens then, jogging will remain a low intensity aerobic exercise. However, most joggers I see on my early morning walks are definitely exercising intensely and consequently burning glycogen and not fat. They are usually overweight, red faced, pouring sweat and puffing and panting fit to burst. They look to be in a really terrible state and I have to resist the temptation to take out my mobile and call for an ambulance.

Reverting to body weight for a moment, it is important to be aware that your overall weight is no guide at all to your body fat percentage. Suppose you weighed 180 pounds when you started resistance training and over the course of the next 3 months managed to put on 5 pounds of pure new muscle, while at the same time losing 3 pounds of body fat, your overall weight would have actually ***increased*** by 2 pounds to 182 pounds. However you would be much healthier as your body fat percentage has ***reduced***, thanks in large part to the new muscle.

So overall body weight on its own is no guide as to how you are progressing in strength training or in losing fat. In fact in the above example, where an individual actually increased in overall weight by adding muscle and losing fat - ie becoming healthier - that same individual's Body Mass Index would have actually increased! The Body Mass Index (BMI) is now quite rightly being consigned to the rubbish bin. It is simply a ratio of body weight to height an makes no allowance at all as to how much of that weight is LBM and how much is just fat. The British army have now stopped using the Body Mass Index in their selection criteria because they were excluding some of the strongest (but heaviest) recruits.

Many people will actually put on weight as they start to get fitter and stronger. In my own case I found that my weight tended to stay around the same 180 pound level over the first few years of training.

However I was definitely getting stronger, lifting heavier and heavier weights, so I knew that my body fat percentage just had to be reducing. In fact my waist measurement was slightly improved (smaller) in confirmation – but even if I had maintained the same waistline I still had to be losing body fat. If you put on new muscle and remain the same weight, then something has to go – and that something, you will be pleased to hear, is fat. So I was building muscle and losing fat pretty much at an identical rate, thus maintaining the same overall approximate body weight. If you are very overweight when you start training it is likely that you will lose initially more fat than the amount of new muscle you build – in which case your weight will drop.

If your goal is to build new muscle, and to lose fat at the same time, then you should definitely concentrate on building the new muscle first, maintaining the same calorie in ignoring your bodyweight completely for the first few Provided you are eating correctly the fat loss will tend after itself. This is because firstly you are burning mo ries when exercising and secondly because the more muscle you build the more calories you are burning while at rest. Your metabolism has been raised.

Once you have built the new muscle then you can reduce your calorie intake slightly to help budge stubborn fat deposits. But only slightly, and gradually, or you risk cannibalising the new muscle that you have worked so hard to build.

A good target for body fat would be 10% for men and 15% for women, who naturally have a higher body fat requirement. Top athletes may get down to 5% and 8% for men and women respectively. But at the levels I suggest you would be in excellent shape. Unfortunately it is difficult to measure body fat reliably. Most gyms use skin fold callipers but these can be unreliable unless the person testing is very experienced. Other ways to measure body fat are by underwater weighing, and various electrical methods where differing resistances to a low current, passed through the body by suitably attached electrodes, are measured.

The good news is that it is not really necessary to have your body fat measured accurately (unless you are in the running for the Mr Olympia title) as it is easy to asses whether your body fat level is in a healthy range once you have been exercising for a few months. Simply keep a record of your body weight, waist measurement and the maximum weight you can bench press for one repetition, known as your 1 Rep Max (1RM). As you will discover in Part 2 you will be encouraged to keep the 1RM recorded anyway. In fact if you are a typical male this is the one number that you will be the least likely to ever forget.

Provided your overall weight is maintained (or increases) while your waistline is maintained (or reduces) then your body fat percentage is constantly improving (reducing) – with the proviso that your strength, as defined by your 1RM is increasing (see Chapter 19 'The Benchmarks of Strength'). The higher your lean body mass (LBM) percentage is, the easier it becomes to reduce the remaining body fat. Build new muscle and you will increase your metabolism. Increase your metabolism and you will burn more fat.

The third benefit of strength training is as equally as exciting as the first two. It will be of particular interest to women whose bones tend to leach calcium, with the resulting onset of osteoporosis and consequent hip replacement, much earlier in life than in the case of men.

Chapter 3

Benefit 3: Grow Stronger, Denser Bones
Reversing Osteoporosis

It is not just muscles, connective tissues, ligaments and tendons that can become stronger with resistance training. When bones are moved by stronger muscles and connective tissue the bones themselves become stronger. When a strain is applied to a bone the body responds by forming collagen fibres which then mineralise forming new bone tissue. This process can take several weeks – but once you start lifting heavy weights it is ongoing. All else being equal thicker, stronger bones are healthier bones.

As we get older our bones naturally tend to get more porous and less dense, thus are more brittle and prone to breaking. Studies have shown that between the ages of 40 and 70 the average man will lose about 15% of his bone mass. Resistance training reverses this process and actually ***adds*** density to bones. This applies to all bones including your vertebrae (backbone) and the heavier the weight the better. One case study showed that a power lifter who could squat more than 1000 pounds had the highest bone density ever recorded in human vertebrae, with absolutely no sign of damage. For the elderly an increase or decrease in bone density can mean the difference between active lifestyles and the permanent disabilities that can be caused by hip fractures and other bone breakages.

Getting plenty of calcium is obviously helpful but on its own will not initiate new bone growth. Also the absorption rate of calcium from supplements is often very low – sometimes as low as 20% - 30% so many people may be getting a lot less than they need to maintain healthy bones.

I believe the best way to obtain your calcium is the same way cows do – from the green stuff, but spinach and similar dark leafy vegetables in our case, rather than grass. In fact I gave up calcium supplements altogether several years ago after my researches uncovered one scientific study indicating that calcium supplements may actually be leaching calcium from my bones! If you ever heard the expression 'expensive urine' I believe that is exactly what my calcium supplements were becoming. Since giving up that particular supplement I have noticed absolutely no change whatsoever except a saving of money, and my bones continue to get stronger. I hasten to add that other supplements, I believe, are not only really necessary but absolutely vital in the world in which we now live (see Chapter 27 'Nutrition').

Year on year I drive (force) my bones to get stronger and denser, by forming more collagen fibres, simply by ensuring they are moved by ever increasing muscle mass. There is just no other way.

Your bones are as equally 'alive' as your muscles but they deteriorate even faster if not used. A few bedridden weeks will guarantee the onset of sarcopenia (muscle loss) but this will pale in comparison to the amount of bone loss that will be experienced – especially in the elderly.

Benefit 4 of strength training, covered in the next chapter, deals with maintaining pain free joints – not as romantic as the benefits already discussed but yet another crucial benefit of increased strength, and again, particularly relevant to the elderly.

Chapter 4

Benefit 4: Form Thicker Cartilage and Protect Your Joints

Joints are simply the places where pairs of bones meet. The ends of the bones are covered in cartilage to stop them rubbing against each other, acting a bit like shock absorbers. To avoid friction they are covered with a membrane filled with a liquid called synovial fluid, which acts as a cushion. If your surrounding muscles aren't strong enough, joints tend to slip out of alignment causing uneven wear and tear on the separating cartilage.

Sometimes the cartilage is worn away in places so that your bones may actually scrape against each other causing intense pain and inflammation. When you build up muscle strength this keeps the joints stable, properly aligned, more flexible and less susceptible to this type of wear. Strength training also increases the thickness of cartilage, which having no blood supply, relies on the synovial fluid to bring in the nutrients. Synovial fluid is generated by exercise. Immobility can destroy it. However, it seems exercise may also regenerate dead cartilage.

Although it may not be a scientific biomarker of ageing, not being able to do painless full knee bends is a sign I associate in my mind with old age, and certainly not a condition I want to suffer from. I did have a slight twinge in my right knee in my early fifties and a sports therapist, while not being able to diagnose it, suggested I try glucosamine chondroitin supplementation.

I understand many people with knee problems swear by these supplements, but they did not seem to make any difference in my case, and they are certainly not cheap. As with all supplements you are never quite sure how much is literally going right down the drain. So I just persevered with strength training instead and the irritation, whatever it may have been, finally disappeared several years ago.

Recently, at age 63, I took up squats, a partial knee bend exercise with a weighted Olympic bar placed across the shoulders, in order to add more variety to my leg workouts. This is a very powerful and demanding exercise and there is no way you should attempt it without instruction from a qualified trainer.

However, the point I am making here is that there is no way you will be ***able*** to attempt it if your joints – both hips and knees – are not in perfect health and working order, as this exercise does place some stress on those joints.

There is absolutely no doubt in my mind that the recovery and present health of my joints, enabling me to perform squats, is directly due to strength training combined with daily brisk walking.

The training has strengthened all the surrounding muscles, and therefore the associated ligaments and tendons, while both the training and walking together, I would suggest, have improved circulation so that all necessary nutrients can be delivered efficiently to the joints. The next chapter, benefit number 5, describes other ways that strength training helps to lessen the potential for injury.

Chapter 5

Benefit 5: Lessen the Potential for Injury

Stronger bones, tendons, ligaments and joints are much less prone to injury than weaker ones. As we saw in the last chapter stronger, evenly developed muscles will keep the joints properly aligned when subjected to stress – whether in everyday life, exercise or sport. The stronger you are the more safely you will lift, in the case of weight training, for example. It is the weak individual fooling around with weights who is far more likely to suffer serious injury.

However, the benefits of strength have a much wider potential for avoiding injury in everyday life. Lifting in one form or another, in the everyday situation, must be responsible for the majority of back injuries. Weight training will ensure the muscles are in a good state to lift and, equally importantly, the lifter will know how to lift correctly so that the back is protected. A general rule is to always try and transfer the weight to the leg muscles. So instead of bending over to pick up a heavy object keep your back flat or slightly arched and your shoulder blades together. Lower the whole body solely by bending your knees, To raise the object simply straighten your legs while still keeping your back flat, exactly as you would when doing 'squats' and you will just about eliminate the potential for back injury, even when lifting very heavy objects.

Back injuries caused as a result of incorrect lifting are probably second only to injuries caused through falling. Here I mean falling over - not from a great height, in which case your level of strength is probably irrelevant.

I should know better by now but I still fall foul of an uneven paving stone on one of the morning walking routes I sometimes take. The leading edge sits about 1 inch above the level of all the preceding flat stones. When my toe catches this edge as I am walking fast I start to fall – my arm instinctively flinging out to protect me from the inevitable crash. Then my other leg powers under me forcing me into a sprint with my upper body in an almost horizontal position, until gradually my legs overtake my falling body and I finally end up in a vertical position again – completely undamaged. All this happens on autopilot as it were but I could not possibly have avoided injury if my legs had not been sufficiently strong. If your legs are not strong enough you will fall and the most likely injury will be to that outstretched arm which will possibly fracture. Interestingly enough, and thanks to very efficient modern safety bindings, most skiing injuries are now reckoned to be broken thumbs rather than broken legs. However, as we have already discovered, the stronger the bone in that outstretched arm, the less likelihood there is of a fracture.

So stronger muscles both help you to avoid injury in the first place, and lessen the impact when injury is inevitable. If a fall is unavoidable it is the person with the stronger bones who is much less likely to suffer a fracture. Moving on to the next benefit, it is universally accepted that high blood pressure is dangerous to health. Chapter 6 shows how strength training can reduce it back to normal levels.

Benefit 6: Lower Blood Pressure

It is well known that high blood pressure is linked to many diseases, including potentially fatal ones such as heart disease and cancer. Many factors contribute to high blood pressure including obesity, diet, stress, smoking, high cholesterol levels, lack of exercise, too much salt, depression and genetics. It is not possible to do much about the latter if you are predisposed to high blood pressure – but you can at least marginalise all of the other factors that are under your control. All else being equal, the older you are, the more likely you are to suffer from high blood pressure, in part due to stiffened arteries. A fit, healthy 75 year old has a higher risk than a healthy 30 year old, albeit still a low risk provided he continues to exercise.

Strength training actually lowers blood pressure both directly and indirectly. The release of endorphins in to the bloodstream following strenuous exercise has a beneficial effect. The consequent mood improvement both improves (removes) depression and lowers stress levels, both contributors to high blood pressure. Lowering cholesterol levels – or rather lowering 'bad' LDL levels while raising the 'good' HDL is also beneficial – which is in turn helped by strength training (see Chapter 8 on the subject of cholesterol).

The average midpoint of the normal range for blood pressure, which is measured as two figures: systolic over diastolic, is 120/75. It is one of the easiest biomarkers of ageing to get checked, and for free. You do not even need to visit a doctor. Any self respecting gym will have the equipment and necessary qualified instructors to check your blood pressure and indeed many will go through this procedure as part of a general health check before letting you lose on the weights. My blood pressure at age 60 was 138/87 within the normal range, but very close to the top end of normal which is 140/90. Now at 65 it is 130/80 I am convinced the improvement is down to exercise, both aerobic and lifting heavy weights, since my diet has hardly changed in that time, and is anyway optimised for muscle growth rather than weight loss – an aid to lower blood pressure. Blood pressure is linked to circulation covered next.

Chapter 7

Benefit 7: Improve Circulation

When your muscles get that pumped up look from lifting heavy weights it is the blood flowing into the muscles that causes it, and seeing it in the mirror causes a similar pumped up feeling in your brain. In short you feel great. You can actually see a few veins under that reducing layer of subcutaneous fat. This is what exercising with heavy weights does; forces blood to every muscle under stress, wherever on your body it is.

The heart is not the only muscle to pump the blood. Whenever any muscle contracts it squeezes blood towards the heart, and when it relaxes it fills with blood again exactly like the heart. Healthy, strong muscles not only take the burden off the heart, they actually support it. I cannot think of a better way to encourage and improve circulation. In my experience aerobic exercise does not have this profound effect – whatever its other benefits may be.

I am a great believer in massage as a means to improve circulation, but have come to look on massage as an optimal means of total relaxation and of draining the lymph system to detoxify the body. A really experienced and talented masseuse will get so many toxins released into your bloodstream, a necessary preliminary to their elimination from your body, that you will feel completely whacked out until that elimination process is complete – usually 24 hours. The same massage will definitely improve circulation to some extent – but how can external third party pressure on a particular muscle, when you are in a relaxed state, compete with your own heart forcing the blood to every fibre of that same muscle when under stress?

Strength training will ensure excellent circulation which is necessary to bring the nutrients and oxygen to the muscles, without which they cannot grow.

Good circulation is also important for the regulation of body temperature, particularly as you grow older. If you have ever had a cold bath, or plunge, in winter you will appreciate how circulation helps your body temperature – by keeping you wonderfully warm for the rest of the day. You should also never suffer from chilblains. But good circulation has far more wide reaching benefits, and particularly for the elderly. It is estimated that over 20 million US citizens now suffer from arthritis in one form or another, and this figure is expected to rise to sixty million by 2020 when the 'baby boomers' generation start turning 60[1]. While good circulation alone may not be able to cure arthritis it will always benefit the condition – and similar conditions such as gout – simply by preventing the build up of uric acid in the joints. In fact there can hardly be an ailment that will not benefit from improved circulation.

Benefit 8 covered in the following chapter ensures your cholesterol ratios remain correctly balanced – a balance now considered vital to optimum health.

[1] Estimates from the Centres for Disease Control and Prevention, Atlanta

Chapter 8

Benefit 8: Reduce 'Bad' Cholesterol (LDL) and increase 'Good' Cholesterol (HDL)

You would have to be living on another planet to be unaware of the constant warnings of the many dangers of high cholesterol levels both in your blood and in the food you eat. In fact cholesterol is a natural and essential substance found in all animal cells and is manufactured by your liver. Having too little can be just as deadly as having too much.

There are two important types of cholesterol to be aware of – Low Density Lipoproteins (LDL) and High Density Lipoproteins (HDL) which function quite differently. The LDL cholesterol is known as the *bad* one, contributing to heart disease by creating a waxy plaque build up in the arteries of the heart. HDL on the other hand, known as the *good* one, has the ability to cleanse plaque and so lower the risk of heart disease.

So whereas it was once your overall level of cholesterol that was counted, your medical practitioner will now be far more concerned about the individual levels, wanting to see the LDL level falling and the HDL in fact rising. It is the ratio between the two types that is all important, and it is this ratio that is one of the scientific biomarkers of ageing.

It is generally considered that the bad LDL cholesterol level should not exceed 60 percent of your total cholesterol. I believe many people are still taking drugs to lower their overall cholesterol levels. As with any drug taking there are going to be side effects – but in the case of cholesterol lowering drugs the side effects have been demonstrated to cause cancer in laboratory animals[2]. The long term side effects could prove to be disastrous – it is just not worth the risk.

Increased levels of the bad cholesterol are far better avoided through exercise and a healthy diet, meaning a diet low in saturated fats and sugar – as opposed to avoiding cholesterol rich foods such as eggs and shell fish. It has always seemed to me to be too simplistic to believe that just eating foods containing cholesterol will automatically convert to in-

---

[2] Drs. Newman & Hulley 'Carcinogenicity of lipid-lowering drugs' *Journal of the American Medical Association (1996) 275:55-60*

creased levels in your body – any more than cows drink milk in order to produce it. I eat eggs in one form or another on a daily basis, and would always opt for boiled lobster rather than a greasy (high saturated fat) shoulder of lamb, believing that the virtually fat free protein of the lobster is less likely to raise my LDL levels than the saturated fat of the lamb.

The good news is that whatever you choose to eat, it is exercise, and specifically strength training it is now appreciated, that actually lowers LDL (bad) cholesterol while at the same time increasing HDL (good) cholesterol – thus correcting your cholesterol ratios.

The next two benefits of strength training naturally increase the body's supply of vitally important hormones.

Chapter 9

Benefit 9: Increase Production of Human Growth Hormone

Human Growth Hormone (HGH) is produced by your pituitary gland in spurts, mostly when you are asleep and reasonably sober, since alcohol interferes with the release of the hormone. Heavy resistance training causes your body to produce more HGH with all the consequent benefits. But the exercises used to manipulate the release of extra HGH in this manner must be vigorous and intensive. Playing around with light weights will not trigger any release of the hormone.

Growth hormone increases your body's production of collagen and cartilage. About one quarter of all of the protein in your body is collagen. Collagen is a major structural protein, forming molecular cables that strengthen the tendons and vast, resilient sheets that support the skin and internal organs. Bones and teeth are made by adding mineral crystals to collagen. Collagen provides structure to our bodies, protecting and supporting the softer tissues and connecting them with the skeleton.

Increased HGH is also known to boost sexual potency, improve your sleep, improve memory, and decrease the wrinkles in your skin! Not so surprising therefore that HGH is known as the elixir of youth – natural HGH that is.

Synthetic HGH is constantly being advertised over the Internet, which is understandable considering its potential for turning back the clock. However, I would strenuously advise readers never to consider this option under any circumstances whatsoever. Firstly you do not know what you will be getting, secondly the cost will be exorbitant and thirdly, even if the product does not actually damage you, it will never ever be a long term solution. If you want to roll back the clock and regain lost years - then yes, HGH is a powerful solution – but get it from your own pituitary gland, as I do, by short bursts of really intensive exercise such as weight lifting. Aerobic exercise will not trigger the release of HGH. The medical profession is reluctantly being forced round to the view that so many of the supposed benefits of aerobic exercise, whose history is littered with corpses, are in fact due to resistance (or anaerobic) training instead.

Chapter 10

Benefit 10: Raise Testosterone Levels

Testosterone can be considered the original anabolic, meaning growth, hormone. It is the hormone primarily responsible for normal growth and development of the male sexual and reproductive organs, including the penis, testicles, scrotum, prostate, and seminal vesicles. It facilitates the development of secondary male sex characteristics such as musculature, bone mass, fat distribution, hair patterns, laryngeal enlargement, and vocal chord thickening. Additionally, normal testosterone levels maintain energy, healthy mood, fertility, and sexual desire.

Testosterone production declines naturally with age. Testosterone deficiency may result from disease or damage to the hypothalamus, pituitary gland, or testicles. Depending on age, insufficient testosterone production can lead to abnormalities in muscle and bone development, underdeveloped genitalia, and diminished virility. Studies have also shown that men with obesity, diabetes, or hypertension may be twice as likely to have low testosterone levels as normally fit individuals. Testosterone deficiency has also been linked to osteoporosis.

While testosterone levels can be artificially increased through hormone replacement therapy (HRT) the side effects of this treatment can be horrific – ranging from liver toxicity and tumours to fluid retention, acne and abnormal breast development. To my mind any therapy that plays around with the body's hormone balance has the potential for disaster – and I think the recent re-evaluation of, and the controversy surrounding, HRT bears this out.

Weight training increases the body's levels of testosterone ***naturally***, which in turn delays the onset of the usual age related symptoms. The more intense the effort the more dramatic the increase in testosterone levels will be. Aerobic exercise, on the other hand, as was the case with the release of HGH discussed in the previous chapter, will actually shut down testosterone production.

So if you wish to retain your virility into advanced old age just get down to the gym and start bench pressing.

Chapter 11

Benefit 11: Improve Insulin Sensitivity

Insulin is another vital hormone that is released into the body by the pancreas. Its role is to enable the glucose in the bloodstream to enter the body's cells to be turned into energy. How much insulin is released is determined by what you eat – which in turn will be converted to glucose. Starchy carbohydrates such as potatoes, pasta and rice will be turned into glucose very quickly.

Other carbohydrates, lower on the Glycemic index, will be processed more slowly helping to avoid blood sugar peaks. Without insulin the glucose cannot enter the cells. However, with too high a level of insulin present in the blood stream the cells stop responding and the glucose cannot get through, resulting in insulin resistance.

Insulin resistance is a loss of insulin sensitivity, so that the cells of the body are no longer sensitive to, and consequently cannot respond efficiently to, the hormone. The pancreas, therefore, has to churn out more and more insulin to have any effect. The resulting higher levels of insulin in the bloodstream cause even more insensitivity etc., etc. creating a dangerous vicious circle. Insulin resistance is linked to disorders such as diabetes, heart disease, arteriosclerosis, obesity and thc inability to lose fat.

Loss of strength lowers your blood sugar tolerance and increases insulin resistance.

Whereas strength training actually improves you body's sensitivity to insulin, making just a little of this hormone go a long way. This not only helps minimise body fat storage, but also prevents insulin resistance. Moreover if you already have some insulin resistance strength training, combined with a reduced sugar diet, will improve your insulin sensitivity to healthy levels. All of which will benefit your immune system as discussed in the following chapter.

Chapter 12

Benefit 12: Strengthen the Immune System

You cannot see your immune system, but it is working around the clock protecting you from invasion by a multitude of bacteria, microbes, viruses, toxins and parasites that are constantly trying to infest your body. It also acts immediately to repair damage from invasion by larger objects that you can see – such as splinters, as well as simultaneously trying to eject them. This is why organ transplants often do not 'take' – because your immune system regards them as foreign bodies and, as such, items to be rejected.

Because your immune system works largely unnoticed it is easy to take it for granted – that is until something goes wrong and it fails for some reason. If you catch a cold it indicates that it has failed temporarily to some extent – but the fact that you get rid of the cold assures you it has now recovered. If your immune system did nothing, you would never get over a cold or recover from anything else for that matter. Another example of the immune system at work is the itchy red bump it forms when you are bitten by a mosquito.

To illustrate the importance of the immune system, all that you have to do is look at what happens to anything once it dies. Its immune system (along with everything else) shuts down, and in a matter of hours the body is invaded by all sorts of bacteria, microbes, parasites etc. None of these creatures are able to get in when your immune system is working, but the moment it stops the door is wide open. Once you die it takes only a few weeks for these organisms to completely dismantle your body and carry it away, until all that's left is a skeleton. It is thus vital to maintain a healthy immune system.

Strength training has an immediate beneficial effect on the immune system - whereas loss of strength increases insulin resistance (as we discovered in the preceding chapter) causes bone loss (see Chapter 3) slows the metabolism (see Chapter 2) and increases the risk of injury. All of these and other decadent states place extra loads on the body's immune system – so that when new threats to health are encountered the immune system is less able to handle them, resulting in lowered resistance to infection. Nutrition is another vital factor in building a strong immune system – as is exposure.

Like muscles, the immune system is subject to the law of Use It or Lose It. If you do not use your muscles they will atrophy, and if you do not need a strong immune system it will weaken – which is fine if you visit a desert island and like it so much you decide to stay there forever. However, should you return to civilisation with its killer diseases, the weakened immune system will immediately become apparent.

A real life illustration of this is the plight of two healthy young researchers who visited a bird sanctuary in the Irish Sea off the coast of Anglesey. The sanctuary took the form of a rock that had never been inhabited and was devoid of any sort of pollution – swept daily as it was by clean Atlantic winds.

The two researchers took all necessary provisions with them and had no human contact until the tug arrived to return them to the mainland at the end of their 6 week project. They went straight to the railway station and within 10 hours were back in London, where they immediately contacted severe influenza. Other complications set in requiring hospitalisation, which compounded the situation further as hospitals are awash with every germ imaginable.

They were both near death for several days before recovering - before their immune systems had re-learnt how to handle the multitude of germs surrounding them. Just 6 weeks in a totally clean, pure environment, devoid of any pollution, had left their immune systems with nothing to do - and if you do not use it nature will assume you neither need nor want it, and act accordingly.

The nurses treating them, on the other hand, were completely immune to infection thanks to the massive daily onslaughts their immune systems were well practiced in handling.

A stronger body will give you a stronger immune system.

Chapter 13

Benefit 13: Diminish the Risk of Heart Disease and Cancer

Heart disease and stroke remain the leading causes of death amongst men in the western world, closely followed by cancer. Being overweight, and unfit, will almost certainly indicate both high blood pressure together with elevated levels of LDL (bad) cholesterol – two of the major causes of heart disease and stroke. High blood pressure (as discussed in Chapter 6) and high levels of LDL cholesterol (as we saw in Chapter 8) are ***both*** reduced by strength training.

Cancer is the second most common cause of death, and general fitness is now being viewed as a possible safeguard against it, along with healthy nutrition. Whatever the ultimate causes of cancer may be, it is generally considered that the activity of free radicals is a major contributory factor.

Free radical activity is best countered in two main ways. Firstly by a strong immune system suitably fortified with foods high in flavonoids, which include the compounds that account for plant pigments, which in turn give them their colour. Flavonoids are naturally occurring in a wide variety of fruits and vegetables and the darker the colour the more there are. Prime examples include blueberries, prunes, raisins, spinach and Brussels sprouts – but don't overlook red wine, tea (both black and green) and dark chocolate containing 60% - 85% cocoa solids which is packed with flavonoids – not to be confused with the sickly, artificially sweetened variety containing a glass and a half of milk – the last thing your body needs.

The second powerful defence against free radical activity is exercise. Any exercise is better than none but prolonged low intensity activity is probably the best of all in this respect. Do you know anyone who walks 4 to 5 miles a day and suffers from any sort of cancer?

Next best has to be strength training with the resultant release of endorphins into the bloodstream. The consequent feeling of euphoria just seems to rule out the possibility of any disease, let alone cancer. It may take decades to prove scientifically, but I believe the relationship between mind and body is so close that when you feel that good you are literally giving your physical body absolutely no option to entertain any disease whatsoever. The combination of the two exercises – prolonged low intensity, together with short burst high intensity, is the best recipe for long term protection against cancer, heart disease and any other ailment for that matter. The worst form of exercise in my experience is prolonged, high intensity, such as running and jogging.

A long time ago a wise and very experienced chiropractor diagnosed that the otherwise inexplicable back pain I suffered was solely due to jogging, and advised me to desist for good. I thought Christmas had come early – did I really never have to go jogging again? I had never looked forward to it anyway and dreaded the pain that always accompanied the final mile or so. Now it seems my instincts, and my chiropractor, were right. Jogging has nearly killed 2 US Presidents (Carter and Clinton), and the keep fit neighbour who persuaded me to start (and who jogged 5 miles twice a day pounding along tarmac Suffolk lanes) can now hardly walk through permanently damaged knee joints.

For literally millions of years we have evolved as hunter gatherers, accustomed to walking several miles every day searching for and collecting food, with the occasional short burst of high intensity activity – like running up the nearest tree when a lion appears on the horizon. A mere 5 thousand years of 'civilisation' is not going to change how our bodies react or respond to stimuli by one iota.

Jogging is ***not*** part of our heritage. The poor guy who ran the original Marathon delivered his message and then dropped dead. The run had literally killed him stone dead, more efficiently than any cancer could have. It is worth remembering that extensive puffing and panting signals just one message - and only one: your bloodstream is no longer able to supply sufficient oxygen to your muscles in order to maintain your present activity. If you persist at the same level then you risk the same fate as our Marathon runner.

The next benefit, discussed in Chapter 14 shows how strength training will make your energy levels soar.

Benefit 14: Elevate Energy Levels

Having more muscle means that every activity throughout the day is less taxing. That in turn means having extra energy to enjoy life more. Any daily task in life requires a specific amount of energy to complete it, regardless of the strength or weakness of the person performing it. If you have just enough energy to complete every daily task by say 6.00pm – and not a drop more – then you will be absolutely exhausted at that point in time, and completely unable to undertake anything else that day. If you have less energy than required to complete those same set tasks, then you will probably have retired to bed at 5.00pm.

However, if over the course of the next three to four months you put on say an extra 5 pounds of pure new muscle, your energy levels will soar. Those same tasks that you were just able to complete by 6.00pm, just before your energy levels ran dry, are now finished with the greatest of ease. More importantly your energy tank is still half full and you will want to utilise it in a thousand different beneficial ways. Anything from gardening, hobbies, swimming, DIY, evening classes or even a part time evening job. Perhaps even more time in the gym, reinforcing this beneficial circle still further. It sounds too good to be true, but it is simply the result of the laws of physics. I started experiencing this particular benefit very early on in my strength training – certainly by the end of the third month. My partner at the time pointed out that we seemed to be going out every night, both to restaurants, and more particularly to those same receptions whose invitations I had previously binned – on the grounds that I was too tired, and wouldn't it be nice to have an early night in for a change?

I am not suggesting that you should follow my example. This is simply how this particular benefit of strength training, namely heightened energy levels, became apparent to me. I now use this extra energy in different ways – including teaching. Whatever your particular desires or aspirations, the extra energy resulting from increased muscle mass can only enhance your chances of achieving them.

Chapter 15

Benefit 15: Enhance Competitive Sporting Performance

Almost all top professional athletes now incorporate strength training as an essential aid to increased sporting performance. For sports such as tennis, football, basketball and skiing it is now virtually mandatory to spend time in the weight room to strengthen the major leg muscles. Obviously in a sport such as downhill skiing your quadriceps (thigh muscles) can never be too big and strong. Indeed they absolutely have to be in order to survive the hammering they will be subjected to. Whereas a sport like tennis, on the other hand, may not require the same large thigh muscles (although the serve and volley player will appreciate them) it is still beneficial to have them. In this case not so much to withstand the hammering as simply to ensure greater reserves of energy (as covered in the preceding chapter). All else being equal, it is the player with the greater remaining energy and strength that will have the advantage when you are 10 all in the fifth set. The player with the strongest legs knows he is not going to run out of energy. His larger muscles simply mean he has more energy left in the tank.

A perfect example of how strength training can improve performance was demonstrated by the world class tennis player Andre Agassi. Following his Wimbledon championship win in 1992 Agassi dropped right down the rankings until he was no longer even in the top 100. His subsequent climb back to the highest levels was helped by many factors including, as he freely admits, redeveloping his body through strength training. He knew that extra strength meant extra stamina - a prerequisite to winning a punishing 5 set match.

But strength training has also been shown to dramatically increase performance in slightly less energetic sports. Golf, for example. Studies by Peter Sisco the co-author of Static Contraction Training have demonstrated how increased muscle mass in 50 year olds (of both sexes) has transferred directly to increased length in their golf drives giving these players a measurable sporting advantage. Having the edge always helps you feel better – as covered in the following chapter.

Chapter 16

Benefit 16: Feel Better

Greater strength gives you greater confidence, which in turn makes you feel better. Just reaching those targets, whether on a daily, weekly or monthly basis, in itself makes you feel good. When you feel good your mood also improves and you become more relaxed and happy. Problems that may have irritated you become trivial. So strength alone is a major contributor to feeling better.

However, more directly, gaining that strength through anaerobic exercise directly influences your mood through the release of endorphins into the bloodstream. Researchers at Duke University Medical School concluded that depressed patients put on a 16 week exercise program showed almost identical improvements to those who were just given antidepressant medication. I do not know how accurately it is possible to measure an exact level of depression, but what I do absolutely know is what a high I get from those endorphins flowing through my body after a heavy weight training session.

I do not get the same high after aerobic exercise, or for that matter any of the other forms of, basically aerobic, sport I practice occasionally. I may feel satisfied and relaxed after swimming, tennis or jogging (which I have now discontinued as I believe walking to be far more beneficial) but the endorphins are definitely not released into the blood stream. The elation is not there - just a pleasant tiredness.

Whereas after a heavy anaerobic workout the muscles are pumped full of blood, the veins expanded and the endorphins flowing freely. Although the particular muscle groups I worked on feel completely devastated (I always lift to failure as this is essential to stimulate maximum muscle growth - as explained fully in Part 2) my overall energy is so much higher at the end of a standard workout of about 45 minutes than when I started.

This is no flash in the pan. I have noticed this effect consistently over 15 years. The changing room of the particular gym I have used for the last 5 years is up 3 steep flights of stairs. Guests I have taken there have remarked that their quads have had enough workout just getting up the stairs! I walk up slowly and definitely feel a slight burn in the thighs by the time I reach the changing room. Returning 45 minutes later, after a heavy workout, I run up 2 steps at a time without a second thought. My body feels as light as a feather.

I feel euphoric – like I can do anything. I have learnt this through experience over the years. I know that however tired I feel, and tempted to miss a workout, I will feel so much better if I go ahead and do it. This knowledge alone keeps me on course. More importantly, I now use this knowledge to help me conquer problems quite unrelated to the gym. It is much easier to sit down and tackle a problem, of whatever nature, if you know you are strong and are feeling light and clear headed.

There is a definite relationship between how you feel and how you view a problem. Scientists are now starting to discover all sorts of examples of how the thought process can actually affect molecules of matter. Something we all use, intuitively and often subconsciously as well, but without knowing how.

One of the first examples I witnessed, and as an amateur poker player appreciated, was in an old Hollywood film about a poker game. I will never forget the actor Edward G Robinson calling a break after a long bad run, going upstairs, taking a shower, a shave, dressing carefully in new crisp clean clothes before returning feeling refreshed – feeling good. Feeling good makes you feel confident. Did his mood affect the cards? Well it now seems it could have. Anyway in one more hand he destroyed his opponent.

If a shower, a shave and fresh clothes can have this effect – think what a body flowing with endorphins can accomplish. So whether your problem is financial, domestic or business related you will find a solution. There is always a solution.

However, you find that solution so much more easily and immediately when your mood is enhanced. I know of no better way to enhance your mood, without fail, than through strength training. An enhanced mood is definitely helpful in appreciating the benefit described next.

Chapter 17

Benefit 17: Heighten Libido

The link between say a finely chiselled calf muscle, toned by strength training, and heightened libido (sexual desire) may at first sight appear rather tenuous, until you appreciate the secondary contributions of many of the foregoing benefits of strength training.

Perhaps the most obvious benefit that will increase libido is benefit #10 ***naturally*** raised testosterone levels – and here I am referring to the male. The more testosterone you have the better you are able to perform and the more often you will want to. Testosterone is, accordingly, one of the most touted hormone supplements on the internet.

But that is just the start. Benefit #7 improved circulation can only but help, and not only the male, in achieving full arousal and maintaining it. Good circulation is just as important to the full arousal of female genitalia. Again benefit #2 which reduces body fat must also contribute to increased libido; secure in the knowledge that you will be able to undertake a greater range of positions. Whether or not you consider love-making to be a sporting performance, benefit #15 will still apply to a greater or lesser extent, as too will benefit #14 elevated energy levels - an important contributor both to heightened libido and to sustaining the actual sexual performance itself far longer than you thought possible.

I cannot claim that looking up to 20 years younger directly heightens the libido, but it may assist in finding a suitable partner to explore the possibilities with.

However, to my mind the most immediate and tangible evidence of heightened libido is the feeling of elation experienced after training with heavy weights – thanks to the release of those endorphins into the blood stream as discussed in Chapter 16. I have noticed recently diverse but knowledgeable advice that you should go straight from the weight room to the dining room – with which I agree absolutely, and explain the reasons for so doing in Chapter 27 on nutrition. If you really want to benefit from that heightened libido then perhaps you should go from the weight room, straight to the dining room, and then straight onto the bedroom.

Apart from the joys of sex, it is perhaps the final benefit, of the 18 benefits of strength training that I have experienced, that will have most impact on the lives of every human being on the planet as they pass the milestones of 70 and 80. Even at age 65 my greatest fear is not diminishing sexual performance, but the loss of dignity in old age.

Despite all the appalling mismanagement of our natural resources, and the myriad pollutants we are daily bombarded with, life expectancy is, incredibly, increasing – both in the western and third worlds.

In order to appreciate and enjoy that longer lifespan it is essential to maintain mobility and physical independence. The 18th and final major benefit of strength training that I have experienced, covered next, will insure your independence – and ensure it forever.

stretch the backbone, combined with leg raises if you wish. You can easily add half an inch or so to your height in this manner, at least temporarily. However, compression is a problem that simply does not arise with the bench press.

It is for these reasons that I have chosen the bench press as the ideal benchmark of strength – and use it in examples continuously throughout the remainder of this book. However, the recommended number of sets and repetitions will apply to almost all of the other exercises.

Likewise, I have chosen the bodyweight as the ideal target weight to aim for. Saying you can lift 100 pounds is completely meaningless if we do not know how big you are to start with. However, being able to lift your bodyweight means you are strong. End of story. If any colleagues question this you can always invite them down to the gym to give it a try.

Obviously to a professional weightlifter or body builder bench pressing their bodyweight will be no overwhelming deal, especially in the lighter divisions. In fact I would expect such individuals to be pressing 150% of their bodyweight. These are very strong men who train professionally for many years. For an average fit individual to be able to bench press his bodyweight requires a level of strength that definitely puts him in the 'strong' category. Certainly strong enough to reap all of the benefits of strength training covered in Part 1 of this book.

Perhaps I should explain that this benchmark of strength (lifting an amount equal to your own bodyweight) did not occur to me in dream, or overnight. It developed over time as I started to become interested in what weight I should be lifting, and indeed what weight I could be lifting, in order to continue reaping all the various benefits of strength training that I was starting to experience.

I think the 'eureka' moment arrived one day in my late fifties when I was lifting with a much heavier, stronger and younger (aged 28) partner. Towards the end of our training session I happened to remark that he was a strong guy to be lifting such a weight. He replied that, on the contrary, I was strong to be lifting the weight that I was able to.

Although we were different body sizes we had two things in common: we both regarded each other as being strong – and we were both lifting just over our bodyweights. At the time I weighed approximately 160lbs and was lifting 180lbs and my partner weighed about 195lbs and was lifting around 215lbs. Despite the difference in the amount of weight being lifted we were ***both*** lifting the ***same*** percentage of our bodyweight (approx 110% in both cases).

Suddenly I had a benchmark of strength. Not super strength – but strength enough to tap into all the benefits of increased lean body mass that I was experiencing. Whilst this may never be able to be a scientifically authenticated benchmark it has proved over the ensuing years to be extremely accurate over a wide range of body weights and types.

This benchmark is also a wonderful guardian for the rest of your life, once you have lifted your bodyweight. For example, suppose that at age 40 you weigh 180lbs and are able to bench press 189lbs (exactly 105% of your bodyweight). Fast forward 10 years and let us say you now weight 200lbs. You should now be able to lift 210lbs (being exactly the same 105% of your new bodyweight). If you cannot lift this weight it is an absolute indicator that your lean body mass (LBM) percentage has deteriorated. In other words that extra 20lbs of weight you have gained is more fat than muscle.

By continuing to bench press your bodyweight, as you grow heavier, you guarantee that your LBM percentage is not deteriorating. On the other hand if you can now lift 220lbs it is an equally sure indicator that your strength has improved – you are now lifting 110% - a greater percentage of a heavier body-weight. That extra weight you have gained is mostly muscle.

In fact this benchmark is still valid even if you cannot lift your bodyweight. If you can only manage say 90% of your bodyweight then just ensure that this same percentage is still achievable for any increased bodyweight that may occur in the future.

To summarise, when you can bench press your bodyweight you are strong – by any standards – and will reap all of the benefits covered in this book. It does not matter how much or how little you weigh to start with – 100, 150 or 200 pounds plus – just set a target to bench press your bodyweight and you will definitely be strong in relation to your size.

Whether or not you go on to lift heavier weights at least make it your goal to bench press your bodyweight so that you can reap all of the 18 benefits covered in Part 1. Use that benchmark to guard your health forever. The remainder of this book is devoted to how to do exactly just that.

Chapter 20

Before You Start

Join a gym. The advantages of joining a gym, as opposed to trying to set up a home gym, are overwhelming – particularly if you have no previous experience of strength training. Even if you have both the space and the money to properly equip a home gym I would strongly advise against this course of action, at least until you have the necessary strength and knowledge to ensure your safety.

For many exercises you will often need the assistance of an equally strong and experienced lifting partner (spotter). Specifically, when bench pressing free weights to failure you will ***always*** need a spotter. Anytime of the day or evening there will be someone suitably qualified around in the gym who will be more than happy to spot for you, whether an instructor or another member. In most situations this will be far more difficult to arrange in a home gym – perhaps to the extent of having to tailor your workouts around the timetable of your spotter. Not a situation conducive to serious training. Other major advantages of joining a good gym will enable you to:

- Experience highly qualified, professional instruction
- Experiment with the whole range of gym equipment and weights
- Benefit from ancillary facilities, e.g. sauna, steam room and spa
- Train with, and benefit from, other members who have similar motivations and goals

I cannot overstress the importance of these 4 advantages – especially to the beginner, at whatever age. You will recall that my whole strength training experience started at age 50 – but it ***only*** started because I joined a gym.

My sons had a few years previously set up a very elementary bench press apparatus in their attic apartment on which we all used to experiment from time to time. Their focus was more on tennis than strength, and with no knowledge or motivation on my part, the weights soon started to gather cobwebs and rust (which I suspect happens in a lot of other home gyms).

It was an instructor in my very first gym who explained to me the many benefits of a major body exercise like the bench press, and encouraged me to become proficient at it. The same instructor taught me the basics of sets and repetitions, and how to set and record increasing targets from week to week.

I still had absolutely no idea how this was benefiting me – if at all – but when about 6 weeks down the line that same instructor remarked on my increased chest size, I was hooked. I still had years of learning and refining technique ahead of me, but thanks to joining that first gym I had the basic knowledge of how to use strength training in order to achieve results – and reap the corresponding benefits. In short I was motivated. I was motivated because I was getting results. I was getting results because I was training with the benefit of professional instruction. This simply cannot happen in a home gym.

In a good modern gym the calibre of the instructors and coaches, both male and female, is extremely high. Typically most instructors will be university graduates; qualified members of NSCA (National Strength and Conditioning Association), ACSM (American College of Sports Medicine) or similar bodies and all will be on the REP (Register of Exercise Professionals). Each instructor's particular area of interest may vary, focussing on one of the many specialist fields ranging from say, sports nutrition through to Pilates or the martial arts. However, all of them will be able to devise a training program tailored to your individual needs and goals. Most importantly all instructors will be able to demonstrate each exercise using the correct form or technique – more on which later.

On a personal level I have never come across an instructor who has not been friendly and enthusiastic. This tendency to encourage, and maybe to raise the bar a little, is extremely helpful when you first start training. Maybe I have been lucky in my choice of gyms – but I think not. Professional exercise and fitness teaching is now a highly desirable career choice for many talented young people. It is consequently a very competitive industry and any instructor lacking the right personality and enthusiasm will just not stay the course.

That is not to say you will always receive identical instructions on the best means to achieve your objective. Young, keen instructors who hold passionate views on the best way to achieve something are inevitably going to give you conflicting advice from time to time. Their views will always be the best as far as they are concerned, as I promise you so will mine, but at the end of the day you have to develop a sense of what really works for you. Nothing can help you develop this sense more than working out in a gym, or several gyms, and watching, working with and listening to instructors and other members.

A typical example is the perceived wisdom as to how to achieve a new 1 repetition maximum personal best (1RM. see Chapter 24). Simply complete 1 set of 8 reps at 50% of the new targeted weight – and then go for it. Well, I tried that way for several years and for me it is a loser. The huge leap of doubling the weight in one go, and to a new maximum amount as well, is too much of a shock to the system – at least to my system. While it may not be a loser for you, I believe I have found a better way that certainly works for me and I suspect that will also work for many of you who are reading this book – as detailed in the following chapters. That said, none of this beneficial experience and knowledge will be available to you working out alone in a home gym. Worse still would be working out in a home gym with some cowboy giving you the wrong, but only available, advice.

The next reason for joining a gym is to be able to experience the vast range of equipment and free weights that it would be impractical to duplicate in a home gym. Impractical both as to the amount of space required and the financial outlay involved.

Taking dumbbells as an example I continually use dumbbells each weighing from 10lbs (lying reverse dumbbell flys) right up to 85lbs (seated incline dumbbell presses) and sometimes more for one-arm bent-over rows. My local gym, catering as it does for both men and women, carries dumbbells ranging in weight all the way from 2 to 100 pounds. That is an awful lot of dumbbells – and of course you need 2 at each weight. I have occasionally come across racks of dumbbells for sale in retail sports shops but have never seen any heavier than 10kg or 22lbs each, which frankly is quite insufficient a weight for an average man for even biceps curls – let alone major body exercises such as dumbbell bench presses.

Then there is the only slightly narrower range of barbells, and the racks to hold them all. The bench press and its associated Olympic bar and supports will not exactly fit into a shoe cupboard – nor will the pairs of weight plates ranging from 2.5lbs each up to 45lbs that will go on that Olympic bar – and you will need 2 sets of the 45 pound plates once you are benching over 250lbs. All in all already a huge amount of equipment.

So far I have considered free weights but that is just the tip of the iceberg. The range of exercise machines is now enormous and their footprints are very large. The best machines use free cables so that natural movement is not restricted at all. Machines with two cable pulleys, allowing both arms to be exercised simultaneously, are the best of all but take up the most space. A smaller but still important consideration is that many of these machines are extremely heavy and once installed will be a problem to move.

The two machines that are most relevant to the bench press are the Smith Machine, illustrated below, and the Power Rack.

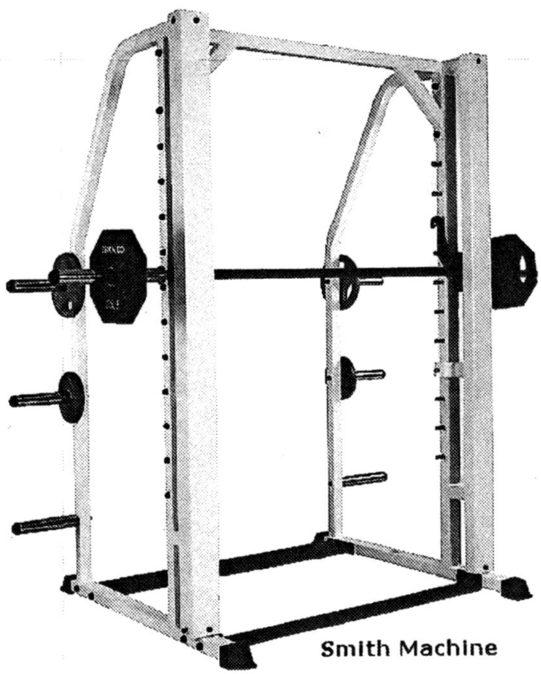

Smith Machine

The main difference is that with the Smith Machine the bar is permanently held by rigid tramlines within which it ascends and descends. Whereas, in the Power Rack (see below) the bar, once lifted off the pins, becomes a free weight.

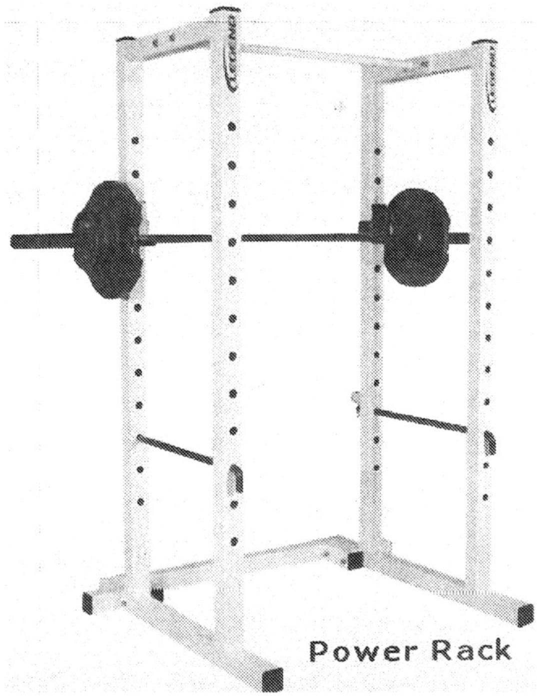

My best advice is to visit a gym and then decide if you really want either of these two giants in your home – that is if you are lucky enough to find a gym in the UK that even has a Power Rack.

The third of the 4 major advantages of joining a gym is to benefit from the ancillary facilities. At the very least these will always include a good shower room and sauna. More usually there will be a pleasant relaxation area, bar and multi channel TV facilities – often with screens directly viewable from the exercise bikes into which you simply plug your earphones. One of the many channels available will be news – CNN or similar

– and it is surprising how useful this becomes in keeping up to date with what is going on in the world while at the same time taking your mind off the drudgery! The bar incidentally is useful for the essential post workout power drink (alkaline, not alcohol based) more on which in Chapter 27 on nutrition.

However, to me the most important of these ancillary facilities is the steam room and spa – but particularly the steam room. To many of my friends it is the sauna. My fair skin has never taken to the sauna and by the time I have been in it long enough to break a good sweat I feel, and look, like a lobster. The minute you enter the steam room, however, your pores open and the sweat just rolls off you. The toxins pour out of you. This is both pleasant and extremely beneficial. The heat is a welcome relaxation after a hard workout, and through your pores you are eliminating both uric and lactic acid, which the workout will have built up in your muscles. Above all you feel really good.

How you feel affects every aspect of your life, physiology and progress to an extent, I believe, far greater than we can yet understand or begin to explain. That does not stop us from experiencing this wonderful state. When you know you are going for broke in the weight room there is nothing more encouraging (to me) than knowing the steam room awaits. The steam room has become to me the carrot and if I am aware it is temporarily out of order I will seriously consider postponing a workout. For carrot perhaps read reward, for there is no stick in the workouts I will encourage you to undertake.

The final advantage of the 4 that I listed above for joining a gym is perhaps the most important of all, depending upon your objectives. For me it has certainly been the most satisfying and rewarding – and that is gaining the enormous benefits of motivation, competitive goal setting and encouragement from a lifting partner – none of which may be available to you in a home gym. I find the continual discussion and evaluation of technique, what weight to attempt, what exercises to do next etc. not only valuable but absolutely essential.

Equally essential are the comments of a lifting partner checking your form, and not just for safety as in the bench press, but in say the case of the cable triceps push down. A partner will quickly point out if your upper arms start to move – and likewise you in turn will be able to correct any bad form on his/her part. Even on days when there are no lifting partners around you will be able to keep check on your position in the full length mirrors which cover the walls of most modern gyms, and for this very purpose.

However, it is in the areas of goal setting and inspiration that I find it most beneficial to have a lifting partner, who will most likely have similar objectives to my own. Having a good lifting, or workout, partner will instil a sense of competition and make workouts much more enjoyable.

More importantly you will be spurred to greater effort and lift weights that you would just not consider attempting on your own. It really helps if your partner is slightly stronger than you, and I would definitely encourage you to try and strike up an acquaintance with any other members of your gym who might at first glance look dauntingly big.

You will be amazed at how quickly you will be able to workout seriously with them, even though you may never truly compete with them at the heaviest weights. That does not matter. I am very fortunate in having met 3 or 4 such individuals with whom I workout fairly regularly. Being the weakest, I am constantly playing catch-up which is great. Great because I am being encouraged to lift weights I would just not otherwise consider - and great because as their targets increase so do mine. I cannot over-emphasise the importance of lifting partners. Unless you are extremely lucky all of these benefits will be denied to you in a home gym.

I used to think that workout partners were not really necessary on what I call the ancillary exercises, such as the biceps and triceps when, at least for safety reasons, a spotter is not required. How wrong in practice I have proved myself to be. In my 64th year both my biceps and triceps maximum weight levels rocketed thanks to performing the relevant exercises with much stronger partners. This is to some extent psychological. There is no big deal about doing preacher curls – and yet one week later, working out alone, I could not achieve the number of reps that I had previously completed when working out with my stronger colleagues.

Once you start lifting heavy weights (anything over 200lbs) psychology will play a part in your performance – a minor part I had erroneously thought in most ancillary exercises – but a very significant part when it comes to major body exercises such as the bench press. That is a fact that you will have to learn to live with - and just accept.

You will have bad days. You will sometimes be as much as 30/40lbs off your 1RM and wonder why. Just take a few days off and recall why you are involved in this whole process anyway. Remember, it is simply to gain the 18 major benefits of strength for the rest of your life. If you follow my advice in the next few chapters you will be continuously gaining in strength, regardless of a one day poor performance.

I say again, when it comes to the bench press psychology will play an increasing role as you graduate to the maximum weights. Psychology, luckily, is a doubled edged sword. On a bad day it will ensure you lift well below what you just know you are capable of – but on a good day it will assist you to lift far more than you ever thought possible.

It is on such days that you establish your new 1RMs. On such days you will be over the moon. It is on days such as this that you will be motivated forever – and you will never give up on increasing your strength, and consequently reaping all the associated benefits, for the rest of your life.

I do not believe those record days such as I describe above can ever be achieved in a home gym. No partners – no incentives – no competition – no energy and no psychology. Case closed. Join a gym.

Chapter 21

Optimal Routines

For me the routine that is going to deliver the greatest muscle gain in the most efficient manner, and the shortest possible time, must include the following elements:

WARMING UP
OVERLOAD
LOW REPETITIONS
BALANCED TRAINING
PROPER RECOVERY
GOOD NUTRITION
SAFE LIFTING, CORRECT FORM & TECHNIQUE

Without heavy weights there will be no muscle gain. That is the absolute starting point of building larger muscles. Good nutrition and the correct number of sets and repetitions will enhance any muscle gain. Proper recovery will ensure muscle growth takes place, and stays in place, avoiding 'plateauing' and Over Training Syndrome (OTS). Balanced training and correct form will ensure you lift the maximum weights in absolute safety.

But there will ***never, ever*** be ***any*** muscle gain unless the muscle is put under increasing stress. Lifting the same weight each time you work out a particular muscle will achieve the same result – nil muscle growth. The stress on the muscle must be progressive, and this can only be achieved through increasing the amount of weight, the number of repetitions or a combination of both.

For example, let us assume that in week 1 the top set (top as in pyramid – the heaviest weight in your routine) of your bench press is 3 repetitions at 200lbs. In week 2 you should either increase the weight to 210lbs and complete the same 3 repetitions ***or*** leave the weight at 200lbs but increase the number of repetitions to 4. In both cases the total load has increased.

As a rule of thumb, when lifting heavy weights, I prefer to increase the number of repetitions week by week until I can just accomplish 6 (but am quite unable to complete 7) at which point I then increase the weight. I will persevere with the new heavier weight until I can once again just complete 6 repetitions but no more – and then again increase the weight – and so on. This lifting routine of progressive overload is a great week-on-week way to increase strength but obviously does not apply when aiming for a new 1RM.

The subject of overload, along with each of the other 6 essential elements listed above, is covered individually in the ensuing chapters.

All 7 elements are not only vital to success, but taken together they form the very core of what this book is about – the practical 'how to' of building LBM in order to reap all the benefits of increased strength for the rest of your life. Follow these practical steps and you will not fail to achieve really spectacular muscle growth, and develop a lean and hard body into the bargain.

Many books I have read on strength and fitness training devote, sometimes several, chapters to building and then maintaining motivation to stick with a training program – often involving copious form filling and note taking. If you follow the simple steps in the ensuing chapters you will achieve immediate results – and if you have never trained before, the results achieved in the first three months can be quite spectacular. If you put an inch on your biceps absolutely nothing is going to keep you away from the gym. You will not need motivation to train - you will need motivation to stay away, to avoid over training! Success, which in our case means continually increasing LBM, is the only motivation you will ever need.

That is my experience and my promise. I am the first to admit that not all exercises are equally as exciting, and if some important appointment came up that meant I had to miss a 'calf raises' gym session I would not lose too much sleep. I would simply incorporate it into my next workout.

However, it would have to be an appointment of really critical importance to keep me away from the gym on a 'bench press day'. All the other exercises are like a supporting cast to this major upper body exercise, and devised and timed to support it accordingly. When bench pressing I will be lifting more weight than I could possibly lift with any other single upper body exercise. I will be lifting well over my bodyweight. I will be engaging all of the body's massive pectoral muscles, the triceps, the front shoulders as well as various stabilising (balancing) muscles in shoulders arms and wrists. I will be, literally, risking death if my spotter should choose to have a heart attack at the wrong moment.

Perhaps it is this added spice of danger that makes the bench press truly the king of exercises. This possibility of danger is yet another seriously compelling reason to join a gym, rather than trying to set one up at home. According to a Men's Health publication no less than 10 people have died in home gyms in the USA while bench pressing.

With every other free weight exercise there is usually a way out if the weight proves too heavy to hold – even if it means just dropping it. With the bench press, however, once that weight is off the pins there is no going back. None. Dropping an Olympic bar with plates (now weighing say 225lbs in total) across your neck is just not an option.

However, perform the exercise correctly, ***always*** with a competent spotter, and you reduce the risk to less than that of crossing a country road at midnight.

Meet or exceed your target weight, particularly for a new 1RM, on a bench press and you will be over the moon. You will be euphoric and your motivation will soar. Nothing will keep you away from the gym. You certainly won't need any notes to remind you what weight you have just lifted. As in any other walk of life, the better you become at achieving something, the more you enjoy doing it. The more you practice it the better you become – a truly beneficent circle. In my experience success is the only motivation you will ever need. If you include all the suggestions in this book in your training routine you are guaranteed to succeed.

The next chapter covers the first of the 7 essential elements listed above and is where you start to get the practical knowledge to enable you to bench press your bodyweight.

Chapter 22

Warming Up

Warming up is an absolutely essential preamble to any workout involving heavy weights. Its object is twofold - both to ensure safe lifting, and to enable you to lift heavy weights. There are two stages to warming up and both are equally important.

STAGE 1

The first stage is designed to raise the core body temperature a few degrees. It is usually achieved by several minutes of low intensity aerobic exercise such as brisk walking, jogging or bicycling - either outside, or in the gym using the appropriate machines. The point is that it must not be too strenuous - no huffing and puffing - and you do not want to be sweating buckets - just slightly damp on the small of your back and the base of your neck. Taking a hot shower is no substitute as this simply raises your skin temperature as opposed to your core body temperature.

Since my gym is a brisk 20-minute walk away, my core body temperature is usually raised a few degrees by the time I arrive, when the base of my neck will be slightly damp with perspiration. Nevertheless I still start off with 5 minutes on the exercise bike.

Again, at such a level that I can still breathe easily, just through my nose, and carry on a conversation without puffing.

For me this means 5 minutes at a level 10 of difficulty, and at a speed of around 85 revolutions per minute. If I have driven to the gym, or the weather is particularly cold, I will increase the exercise bike warm up time to 10 minutes to compensate. The point is to ensure the back of my neck is still slightly damp before I move onto the weights, thus confirming I have raised my core body temperature sufficiently.

If you have not done much aerobic exercise recently, or are particularly out of shape, it may initially take a little longer to break sweat, but this will happen more quickly as you get slightly fitter. Raising core body temperature is vital to avoiding injury and you must not skip this stage. Once warm you can proceed straight away to the weights - and stage 2.

STAGE 2

The second stage of warming up is designed to get the blood flowing through the muscles that are going to be put under stress. It is equally as important as stage one - if not more so in so far as lifting heavy weights is concerned. It is through skimping on this stage that I have damaged my shoulder in the past, resulting in a 6-month layoff – so please be warned.

Since I always start with the bench press if this is an upper body workout day, I will use that exercise as an example. The routine applies to just about every other major body exercise you may choose, whether upper or lower body, whether using free weights or machines.

For exercises that just target specific muscles such as biceps or triceps the number of warm up reps indicated below may be halved. As you progress through a workout the remaining muscles waiting to be exercised will require less warming up once major body exercises have been completed.

Now is the time to do any stretching you want to do which should focus on the pectoral muscles in this instance. I tend to use the pec-deck machine with very light weights and a wide angle of movement to stretch my pectoral muscles. I feel this type of stretching is more appropriate to warming up than static stretching - where the muscle is simply stretched against an immovable object and the position held for several seconds. In fact I have come across studies indicating that static stretching will actually slightly reduce the amount of weight that you will be able to lift. The exact opposite of what we are aiming for. I believe static stretching will be much more beneficial ***after*** the workout. After the muscles have been subjected to massive contraction is the best, and surely most logical, time to subject them to static stretching – not before.

Whatever amount of weight I am eventually aiming to bench press I ***always*** start with 20 repetitions of the empty bar.

This is to get the blood flowing into the muscles that are going to be used and to get into a rhythm while practising correct form. The bench press equipment is covered in more detail later on but a quick word about the bar. The Olympic bar used in the bench press weighs exactly 20 kilograms and this is a global standard. The equivalent weight in pounds is therefore just over 44lbs. However for practical purposes most people, myself included, will consider it weighs 45lbs.

All the plates that are loaded onto it are in weights that are divisible by 5 and it is much easier to add up and keep track of the total weight if you take the bar as weighing 45lbs - rather than weighing a fraction over 44lbs. So 45lbs is, accordingly, the weight used in this book.

My fist warm up set therefore looks like this:

SET 1	20 Reps	
	Olympic Bar (empty)	= 45lbs

I then load a 35-pound plate each end to give some weight and to alert my muscles as to what they are going to have to do. So my second warm up set looks like this (note number of reps reduced to 12):

SET 2	12 Reps	
	Olympic Bar	= 45lbs
	Plus 2 x 35lb Plates	= 70lbs
	Total Weight	= 115lbs

I will then replace the 35-pound plates with 45-pound plates but again reduce the number of repetitions, so the third set will look like this:

SET 3	10 Reps	
	Olympic Bar	= 45lbs
	Plus 2 x 45lb Plates	= 90lbs
	Total Weight	= 135lbs

At this point you can safely consider that stage 2 of the warm up is completed and you can now proceed to load whatever weights you want depending on your desired outcome. The object of using comparatively light weights in the warm up is to conserve your strength and energy for the serious lifting that your muscles are now fully primed for.

You can adjust the weights downwards depending on your bodyweight and experience. These are the weights I use at my bodyweight of around 83 kilograms (183lbs) but you would be ill advised to increase them, whatever your strength. Remember this is only a warm up - and the more muscle you have the more important is it for that muscle to be fully primed to avoid injury. You will see experienced 300 pound lifters starting with just the empty Olympic bar, although they may skip either of the warm-up sets and go straight to half the maximum amount they intend to lift, as I occasionally do.

More usually I will do a fourth warm up set (this is really more of a rude 'wake up' set to the muscles rather than a warm up if I am aiming for a new 1RM) with the 45-pound plates plus the 25-pound plates. I may try for 3, 4, 5 or 6 reps at this weight depending on my final target. So this 'wake up' set will look like this:

SET 4	X Reps	
	Olympic Bar	= 45lbs
	Plus 2 x 45lb Plates	= 90lbs
	Plus 2 x 25lb Plates	= 50lbs
	Total Weight	= 185lbs

You may rightly think that as I am now already bench pressing my bodyweight this can hardly be considered a warm up set. I agree - but neither is it (for me) a full-bloodied building set which is going to build new muscle. I do a fourth set for the following reasons (discussed further in the next chapter on overload):

I am lifting a weight I have lifted many times before.
I am not therefore overloading.
I am not lifting to failure.
I am not engaging all muscle fibres.
I am not sweating hard and panting which I certainly would be on a proper 'building' set.

Perhaps it is better to refer to sets 3 and 4 as 'climbing' sets, as set 3 definitely completes the pure warm up, achieving both proper core body temperature + sufficient blood in the muscle group to be trained.

However, as I said right at the beginning of this chapter, the warming up procedure, as well as ensuring safe lifting, will also assist you to lift the heaviest possible weight. There is one ingredient still missing - that is assuming you are hell bent on increasing your 1RM (which I highly recommend you attempt every 12 weeks or so). That missing ingredient is adrenaline.

For several years in my early sixties I could never understand why my maximum strength seemed to appear only after I had been lifting for about 45 minutes, by when most of my lifting partners were ready to finish. In fact it got to the point that I had to start my warming up 30 minutes before my partner even arrived at the gym if we wanted to synchronise our workouts.

I also noticed that set 2 of my warm-up (see above) always hurt my shoulders a little and made me think "boy, I am really feeling weak today if it hurts lifting this small weight", whereas set 3 was definitely much easier to lift – despite being heavier. Also by set 3 any pain in my shoulders had disappeared. At the end of set 4 I felt then, and still do, that I was really firing on all cylinders and ready for anything (remember each repetition of set 4 is approximately my bodyweight). Just a few minutes earlier I had experienced some pain and weakness on a much lighter set! The answer is the missing ingredient – adrenaline.

The adrenaline had started to kick in. If you want to go for a new personal best you need to get your body on fire. You need to really psyche yourself up. You need a lifting partner who will help you in that process. Above all, you need to get the adrenaline flowing.

Unfortunately you cannot turn adrenaline on like a tap. Adrenaline is a hormone similar to testosterone in that certain conditions have to be in place before it is released into the bloodstream. Danger, fear, and stress can all trigger the release of adrenaline. I am sure most readers will be familiar with that rush of adrenaline following a near miss in a car accident, or any other type of accident for that matter, that has the potential for real danger. It is nature's way of priming the body to take massive avoiding action. For millions of years this simply entailed running like hell and climbing the nearest tree.

However, it is not necessary to let a lion loose in the gym in order for you to benefit from the effects of adrenaline. Simply put your muscles under stress. Put them under ***real*** stress, but not for such a length of time that you wear them down. That is exactly what set 4 above does for me. It is a real 'wake up' set.

Earlier in this chapter I said I may do 3, 4, 5 or 6 repetitions of this fourth set for a very good reason. I am trying to shock my muscles sufficiently in order to trigger the release of adrenaline. I am priming them for a heavier weight to come. That is all.

What I am certainly ***not*** trying to do, in this particular instance, is to lift to failure. Consequently I will stop as soon as I feel the speed of the repetitions slowing down - as soon as I feel my energy draining too fast. This can vary from day to day - as will, therefore, the number of repetitions.

There is a very fine line between putting your muscles under enough stress to release the adrenaline - and putting them under such stress that you burn up too much energy in the process. However fit you may be at the start of a workout you have a finite amount of energy. You have to leave enough in the tank to scale that new height - that new 1RM. Finding out ***exactly*** where to draw that fine line is an ongoing process. The line will probably move as your experience, strength and also possibly your age increase. If you follow my own example sets as discussed in this chapter (with the weights adjusted for your own size and capabilities) you will find out where to draw your own 'fine line' fairly easily after a few weeks experimentation.

I am writing this book at the age of 65 with the benefit of 15 years continuous experimentation and experience. I am the living proof that age has absolutely no effect whatsoever on either the rate or amount of muscle growth that can be achieved - but it may possibly have an effect on the speed at which adrenaline is released. This would account for the fact that it seems to take me about 45 minutes in the weight room before I am fully fired up for that new 1RM.

Before leaving the subject of what is the first of the seven vital elements that I would include in any optimal routine - warming up - I would like to suggest one specific exercise that I recommend you include. If you are going on to do the bench press, or any other exercises involving the shoulder muscles, then it should definitely be included.

Although this exercise can be practiced in its own right as part of a regular workout, I use it here purely as part of stage 2 of a warm-up. The object is to get the blood flowing through a group of small but vital muscles in the shoulder that assist with its rotation. They are known as the rotator cuff muscles.

To perform the exercise adjust the height of a pulley on a cable machine to about waist height and adjust the weight to one of the lightest in the stack (about 3 or 4 down from the top in my case). Use a D handle on the cable. Grab the handle and move a few feet away from the machine standing at right angles to it. Bring your upper arm close to your side, keeping it perpendicular with your body, and make your lower arm parallel with the floor. Now rotate the lower arm through 180 degrees while keeping the upper arm absolutely stationary - see the illustration below.

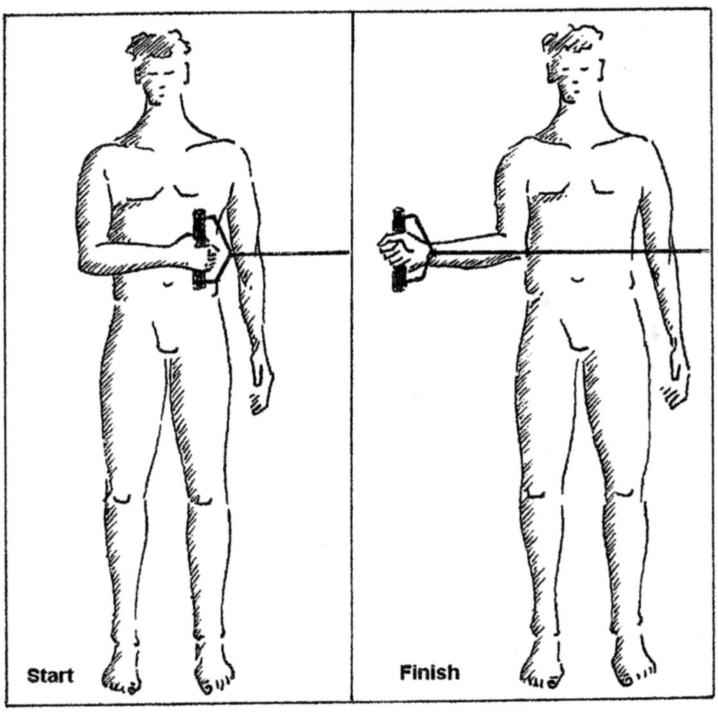

Note that the arm is pulling the weight ***away*** from the body rather than towards it.

To best target the rotator cuff muscles make sure the upper arm stays glued against the body (there is a natural tendency for the elbow to lift away). I usually start with 20 repetitions with each arm then increase the weight and do another set of say 15. I may then increase the weight again and complete a further 10 repetitions. I usually intermingle these sets with my main warm up sets on the bench press. If this seems a lot of repetitions please remember I am using really light weights. I am simply trying to warm up the blood in these specific, small but very important muscles.

The rewards of incorporating this particular exercise in my warm up routine have been enormous to me, as I believe they will be for many others. Specifically I no longer feel any pain in my shoulders when performing the bench press warm up sets. Furthermore I am convinced that if I had been aware of this exercise when I first started bench pressing I would have avoided the shoulder injury and consequent layoff that I experienced (see Chapter 28).

Incidentally this exercise was introduced to me by a young Spanish instructor. Another compelling reason for joining a gym as discussed in Chapter 20. You are not going to be exposed to experienced advice and really helpful tips like this when training alone in your home gym.

Finally, before moving on to discuss heavy weights or 'overload' in the next chapter, I cannot overstress the importance of proper warming up. A few stretches is just not sufficient if you are going to lift heavy weights.

Perform both stages of the warm up as outlined above however, and you are well on the way to lifting both safely and successfully.

Chapter 23

Overload

The 18 major benefits discussed in Part 1 derive directly and exclusively from greater strength. Greater strength comes solely from more powerful muscles - so increased muscle mass or LBM is our goal.

Muscles control your whole physiology. Every movement you make in life from the twitch of a finger to a massive high jump may initiate in the brain – but no part of you can move unless some muscle or other contracts. If someone cannot move their legs it has nothing to with bones, tendons or joints. It is solely that for one reason or another their muscles cannot contract.

Maybe they are paralysed so the brain simply cannot get the message through to the muscle because the nerve chain is broken. Maybe the message got through but the muscles have atrophied to such an extent that they are too weak to move the bone. Maybe it is just too painful to want to contract the muscle.

Whatever the reason, no movement will take place unless the muscle contracts. Muscles are attached to each end of the relevant bone by tendons. If you want to move that bone the brain sends a message to that muscle to contract (when its reciprocal muscle will expand). This contraction of muscle is the ***only*** thing that moves the bone. If no contraction takes place that bone will just not move – except under the force of gravity.

If, standing upright, with your arms hanging at you sides, palms forward, you decide to raise your forearms in front of you until they are parallel with the floor, the movement is principally the result of your biceps contracting, or shortening. (In reality other small supporting muscles become engaged but for illustrative purposes we will stick to the major ones).

Your biceps are attached to bones in your shoulder at the top end and to the radius (forearm bone) at the bottom end. If they contract your forearms have no option but to rise. If you now grasp a dumbbell in each hand and repeat the above movement, but this time raising your forearms further so that they end up closer to your shoulders (about 45 degrees from parallel), you are effectively performing a biceps curl. You may want to start doing this exercise first with one arm and then with the other before going on to curl both biceps simultaneously. You will definitely want to start with light weights - perhaps light enough so that you can complete 15 to 20 repetitions without busting a gut. In other words a typical warm up set which allows you to concentrate on performing the exercise correctly (with good form). In the case of the biceps curl that means checking that your wrists are straight, that you are not swinging the dumbbells up and that your upper arms remain absolutely stationary, against your equally stationary body.

Every successful repetition you complete is the result of your biceps muscle contracting - nothing more. Congratulations. You have completed 1 full set of 20 repetitions of the biceps curl. You may want to rest for a few minutes and then do another set - and then another. The point is you can do this exercise (or any other) with the same light weights, every day for a week, a month or even a year. You can go home thinking you had a good workout but your biceps will not grow one jot. You have exercised the muscle but you have not put it under stress. The ***only*** way to stimulate muscle growth is by subjecting the muscle to stress. That means overload.

You may have watched Marathon runners from time to time. Runners who train (i.e. exercise) their calf, thigh and other muscles on a daily basis. People who run for hours on end often covering 10, 15 or 20 miles at a time. Yet their legs are like matchsticks. Their muscles are painfully thin and they often collapse. In fact the original Mr Marathon man, as we saw in Part 1, not only did just that but then died into the bargain.

It is not of course the runner's objective to build muscle. The Marathon runner's sole objective is to cover exceptionally long distances in record time. The goal is stamina, not strength. It is, however, a good example of how "exercise" in itself will have ***no effect whatsoever*** on muscle growth, strength or size.

The Marathon runner does not care. The sprinter, however, cares very much. The sprinter needs massive legs to power him over a very short distance in around just 10 seconds. Stamina here is irrelevant. Strength is absolutely vital - which explaims the huge size of your average sprinter's thigh muscles.

There are plenty of ways to optimise muscle growth but there is only one way to stimulate it in the first place: overload. If you do not subject your muscles to overload the best training and nutrition in the world will not put on one ounce of extra muscle – nor therefore strength.

It may do all sorts of other things but it will not increase your strength. I am assuming you have read this far because you are excited about the incredible benefits of strength training and want to achieve a biological age at least 20 years younger than your chronological age. Because you want to be strong like our sprinter – not an ambulance case like our Marathon runner.

In this case the fastest, most efficient way to put on muscle is overload. Lift the heaviest possible weights, and lift to failure. This way is the kindest to your joints - much fewer wearing sets and repetitions (see the following chapter).It is also kindest to your busy diary - less time spent in the gym - and best indulges your impatience. By overload I mean both lifting to failure ***and*** progressively increasing the weight being lifted and/or the repetitions being attempted - so that you end up lifting heavy weights. ***This is the very heart of the matter if you wish to put on the maximum amount of muscle in the shortest possible time.*** Anyone who skips this chapter or fails to understand the relationship between overload and muscle growth will be missing (at best) the shortest path to their goals. At worst they will never achieve them.

Overload is the only one of the seven elements that will produce muscle gain. If you ignore the 6 other elements you will still gain some muscle though nothing like the amount you could by including all 7 elements in your routine.

However, exclude overload and you will gain no significant muscle at all. What I term overload comprises using heavy weights, progressively increasing those weights and lifting to failure.

Overload is so important that I will expand on the three ingredients individually:

1) Heavy weights

The word heavy is of course relevant. Relevant to your size and strength. What is heavy to me may not be heavy to you - and vice versa. In the context that I now use it, the word heavy means a weight so heavy that you cannot complete 7 repetitions of an exercise. You may be able to just squeeze out 6 repetitions, but no more. The specific weight is of course also relevant to the particular exercise itself. The same weight that is heavy, according to my definition, for a biceps curl would be no more than a warm up weight for a bench press.

Lifting light weights, as in the earlier example of the 20 repetition sets of the biceps curl, will not increase muscle mass one iota. Neither will running 20 miles. There is a very good scientific reason for this. Muscles are made up of two very different types of fibres called Type I and Type II which are more commonly known as slow-twitch and fast-twitch fibres.

Fast-twitch are the very powerful fibres capable of rapid contraction but which tire easily. Slow-twitch fibres cannot generate the power but have much more endurance. If you lift weights heavy enough so that you can only manage a few repetitions, you recruit the fast-twitch fibres. The greater the effort required the more fibres of both types will be recruited. Lifting light weights will only recruit the slow-twitch fibres – ***and it is the fast-twitch fibres that must be mobilised to achieve muscle growth.***

You must therefore use heavy weights at some point in your workout, and must accordingly aim for fewer repetitions.

I have noticed so many people over the years in various gyms who never seem to change shape. Year in, year out, they exercise to exhaustion, 3 days a week like clockwork, but never grow any bigger. Part of the reason, as we shall see in Chapter 26 on recovery, is overtraining - but a far larger part of the reason is failure to use heavy weights.

These people seem to delight in the number of repetitions they can push out. Typically they perform 3 sets of 12 repetitions each at the same weight. After 36 repetitions they are quite naturally fairly exhausted and reckon accordingly that they must have had a good workout. In fact the weight being attempted was not heavy. The fast-twitch fibres were therefore never engaged - and the result is absolutely nil muscle growth. I promise you. I have been there.

Taking just one of these sets as an example, using say a weight of 100lbs: completing 12 repetitions means lifting 12 x 100lbs = 1200lbs. Quite a large total weight which you may assume should produce at least some muscle growth - but it won't. It won't because the individual lifts were never heavy. You could and should, however, try increasing the weight to 200lbs and reducing the number of repetitions to just 6. The overall total being lifted still remains at 1200lbs but now the weight is heavy. The fast-twitch fibres will become engaged and muscle growth will be triggered.

Heavy weights are an absolutely essential ingredient in any workout aimed at seriously increasing LBM.

2) Progressive increase

Progressive increase simply means that you have to increase the weight month on month if you wish your muscles to increase likewise - month on month. You may think this second ingredient of overload is just common sense - in which case you would be surprised at the number of people who seem to leave their common sense in the locker room. Our friends banging out their 3 sets of 12 repetitions at 100lbs each are not only ever lifting ***heavy*** weights - they are also never lifting ***heavier*** weights. They stick at the same 100lbs!

Mother Nature is an immaculate guardian of her bounty. If you do not use it you really do lose it - on the basis I believe that if you do not use it Nature perceives that you no longer need it. This is presumably why we lost our tails. Nature works equally efficiently over a short time frame. Spend just 2 weeks in bed and see what happens to your leg muscles. In the same way that the body cannot discriminate between a self inflicted diet and a genuine famine, Nature seems to care not why you are in bed for 2 weeks. It may not be your fault, but your leg muscles will just as surely atrophy, whatever the reason.

So while heavy weights are important, progressively increasing them is equally as important. It really is just common sense. What was a heavy weight for you 4 weeks ago will no longer be a heavy weight (for you) after a few workouts when your muscles have grown stronger - so you just increase the weight until, once again, it becomes heavy for you.

3) Lifting to failure

The third ingredient of overload, lifting to failure, ensures that your muscles are 'torn down' which is a necessary precursor to any growth. By lifting to failure I mean commencing a further repetition that you know you will not be able to complete unaided. (This is where a good spotter is absolutely vital in the bench press as you will not be able to press the final rep back up without his assistance).

The reason for this is to ensure that you have engaged every single last fibre that you possibly can. To ensure that there really is nothing left in the tank. The resultant 'damage' is in fact quite natural and healthy and amounts to microscopic tears in your muscle fibres which will then, and only then, grow back bigger and stronger.

If they never get torn down in the first place, the body will not perceive any good reason to make them stronger. Lift weights to failure, however, and the brain will send a message to the muscles to the effect that they better get stronger, and fast, to cope with the new emergency situation that is developing.

So to benefit from overload you must incorporate heavy weights into your workout. You must ensure you progressively increase those weights, and you must lift to failure. Suggestions as to when and how to do this are covered in the following chapter.

Chapter 24

Sets & Repetitions

Sets and repetitions (reps) are the means by which you manage your workout to ensure that you train in the most effective manner.

A repetition is one complete movement of an exercise. A set is comprised of a number of repetitions of an exercise which are performed continuously without pausing. A set may consist of any number of repetitions but typically the number will vary from 1 through to 20. The key to success is in managing both the number of sets, and the number of repetitions within those sets - as well as the amount of weight being moved during each repetition.

As a general rule the number of repetitions will reduce, and the amount of weight will increase, as you progress through the various sets of an exercise. This can progress on occasions until you are attempting a set comprising just 1 repetition at the maximum weight used in that exercise. This would happen, for example, when you are attempting a new 1RM. The weight is now so heavy that you are only able to complete one repetition properly.

Before you commence any exercise decide how many sets you want to complete and then how many reps each set will contain. Both will depend upon your experience, your goals and your particular favourites. The number of combinations of sets and reps is limitless – but they all fall into the level, rising or pyramid categories. You will soon find out what works best (i.e. achieves results) for you.

Every gym instructor will be happy to give you a starting program – and every starting program will be slightly different depending upon that instructor's particular preferences. What follows are examples of what I find particularly work for me. These examples will probably work equally well for most people, but nothing is set in stone.

The number of both sets and reps can be adjusted to suit your own abilities. All I would suggest is that however you may adjust my combinations of sets and reps, you do not leave out 'overload'. Also always aim to end the exercise doing a low number of repetitions of heavy weights rather than the other way around. Given the choice of lifting 1000lbs over 1 set always opt for 5 reps of 200lbs rather than 10 reps of 100lbs.

Firstly, an example of level sets on the bench press could be 3 sets of 8 reps each at the same weight of say 170lbs. A rising combination would involve the same 3 sets but this time the weight is increased for each set. The first set is performed with the same weight of 170lbs but the weight is now increased to 180lbs for the second set – and again to 190lbs for the third set. The number of reps in each set may remain at 8 or may reduce as the weight increases.

A really powerful way to perform this combination is to load such a weight that you can only just complete 8 reps in the first set with correct form. Increase the weight for the second set and lift to failure, maybe completing only 6 reps this time. Rest - then increase the weight yet again for the third set and again lift to absolute failure. You may only manage 4 reps in this final set but I promise you that the results will justify the effort. You are on the road to spectacular increases in muscle strength.

A pyramid combination is as above but instead of stopping at 3 sets you perform a few more but now with a reducing weight. For the fourth set therefore you may reduce the weight back down to 170lbs and perform as many reps as you can. Some would then reduce the weight again to 150lbs for a fifth and final 'cool down' set and knock out say 12 reps.

Others may want to insert a fourth set at 200lbs, at which weight they may only manage 1 or 2 reps before descending the pyramid. As you will see below I tend to workout using pyramid combinations, but all combinations can be equally effective. However, before going on to describe a specific example of my own bench press workout, this is a good point at which to discuss the equipment.

It is possible to perform a bench press using an Olympic bar and free weights or by using a Smith Machine. It is also entirely possible to perform this exercise within a Power Rack although few people may have access to one. However, most gyms will have a Smith Machine. The main advantage of using a Smith Machine is that you can bench press quite safely, including lifting to failure, without the use of a spotter, as safety stops can be placed at regular intervals. When using the Smith Machine for bench pressing I place the safety stops so that the bar is about 3 inches above my chest. Apart from anything else this margin allows me enough space to manage an undignified wriggle out from under the bar when I have lifted to failure!

The main disadvantages of using a Smith Machine are that you are pressing the weight up in an absolutely rigid (as opposed to natural) straight line. Also there is an unavoidable tendency to push against the solid tramlines (that form the rigid frame) thereby gaining some support for the bar which is not of course there when you come to use the Olympic bar - just thin air to push against.

Another small annoyance to me is that it is difficult to measure the exact weight of the counter balanced bar on the Smith Machine, which will vary from machine to machine. I once asked three different instructors in the same gym what the bar on their Smith Machine weighed and received three different answers.

As with most other exercises, if you have a choice always choose free weights over machines – and always include dumbbell exercises in your workout if you bench press or use barbells a lot. When using dumbbells not only can the arm move in a totally natural curve but you ensure that each arm is growing equally strong without any support from the other. With any bar, including the Olympic bar, a weaker arm is able to draw some support from the stronger one through the bar.

The free weight bench press equipment consists of an Olympic bar, a supporting stand, a standard bench and a load of free weights (plates) – also hopefully with their own rack or stand. As mentioned earlier the Olympic bar is a steel bar weighing exactly 20 kilograms, or for the purposes of this book 45 pounds. The plates that you load onto the bar may be marked in either kilograms or pounds. If the latter the plates will range in weight from the smallest up as follows: 2.5lbs, 5lbs, 10lbs, 25lbs, 35lbs and 45lbs.

A little gym speak may not come amiss here. Certainly in some gyms the smallest plates are referred to as the 'biscuits' which they closely resemble. The 45 pound plates are often referred to simply as 'the plates'. So when I say to my spotter that I want to load 'the plates' now it means I am going to load two 45 pound plates each end of the bar - giving a weight of 2 x 90lbs plus the 45lbs for the bar making 225lbs in total.

If someone says he can complete 5 reps with 2 plates it means he can achieve 5 reps of 225lbs each. If you hear someone say he can 'bench 3 plates' it means he can bench press at least 1 rep of 315lbs (i.e. the Olympic bar plus 3 x 45 pound plates each side) and he will probably look the part as well. This must be pretty close to the top weigh for an amateur. To put this amount of weight in context I believe the world record for a single bench press is well over 600lbs, and Arnold Schwarzenegger used to knock out reps of 450lbs[3] on Venice beach.

I have been using pounds in most of my examples but these are easily converted to kilograms using the table of bench press equivalent weights on the next page. Some gyms will have plates and weights denominated in either pounds or kilograms - while others will use a mixture of both, when hopefully there will be a conversion table conspicuously displayed.

Assuming you weigh less than 220 pounds, which most people do, then the next natural target after you have bench pressed your bodyweight is the nice round figure of 100 kilograms. Having achieved that I swap back to pounds for my next target of 225lbs or just 'the plates' - another nice target that is easy to remember.

Thereafter I increase the weight in very small steps. At this level every extra pound is close to that straw that broke the camel's back. However, even increasing the weight by just 5lbs a month still results in a massive annual increase of 60lbs.

---

[3] Encyclopaedia of Modern Bodybuilding - *Simon & Schuster*

BENCH PRESS WEIGHT EQUIVALENTS

Olympic Bar	=	45lbs		
2 x 35lb Plates	=	70lbs		
Total	=	115lbs	=	52kg
Olympic Bar	=	45lbs		
2 x 45lb Plates	=	90lbs		
Total	=	135lbs	=	61kg
Olympic Bar	=	45lbs		
2 x 45lb Plates	=	90lbs		
2 x 10lb Plates	=	20lbs		
Total	=	155lbs	=	70kg
Olympic Bar	=	45lbs		
2 x 45lb Plates	=	90lbs		
2 x 25lb Plates	=	50lbs		
Total	=	185lbs	=	84kg
Olympic Bar	=	45lbs		
2 x 45lb Plates	=	90lbs		
2 x 25lb Plates	=	50lbs		
2 x 5lb Plates	=	10lbs		
Total	=	195lbs	=	88kg
Olympic Bar	=	45lbs		
2 x 45lb Plates	=	90lbs		
2 x 35lb Plates	=	70lbs		
Total	=	205lbs	=	93kg
Olympic Bar	=	45lbs		
2 x 45lb Plates	=	90lbs		
2 x 35lb Plates	=	70lbs		
2 x 5lb Plates	=	10lbs		
2 x 2.5lb Plates	=	5lbs		
Total	=	220lbs	=	100kg
Olympic Bar	=	45lbs		
2 x 45lb Plates	=	90lbs		
2 x 45lb Plates	=	90lbs		
Total	=	225lbs	=	102kg

One final point before leaving the subject of bench press equipment is the use of clips, or other types of stops, designed to prevent the plates sliding off the bar.

These may take the form of either wire spring clips or metal cuffs that are slid onto the bar after the plates have been loaded. I find them to be essential on the short EZ preacher curl bar, as weights are constantly sliding off while loading one side, picking it up and even while performing curls, as it is difficult to keep the hands, and therefore the bar, exactly level.

However, these considerations do not apply to the much longer and heavier Olympic bar used for the bench press. Due to the width of the supports you can load plates quite safely from either side without unbalancing the bar.

Consequently I never used to bother with stops and now I will never bench press with any form of stop on the bar. Not having the plates secured to the bar saved me from serious injury several years ago before I had learnt the hard way about Over Training Syndrome (OTS) as I describe in detail in Chapter 26 on recovery.

EXAMPLE 1

So now on to the first example of one of my typical bench press workouts. The bench press obviously forms part of an upper body workout - and being a major body exercise I always start with it first before exercising the individual muscles such as the triceps and biceps. Whatever my aim for a specific workout I will always start with the 3 warm up sets exactly as described on page 55.

Again, as explained in the chapter on warming up, I will intermingle these sets with the rotator cuff exercises in order to increase the blood flow through my shoulders. So to recap, my third warm up set will be 10 reps of:

Olympic Bar	= 45lbs
Plus 2 x 45lb Plates	= 90lbs
Total Weight	= 135lbs

and any variation in my bench press exercise will only start after this third set has been completed.

At this point I usually put on some lifting gloves. These are entirely optional but I find gloves make lifting much more comfortable. Wearing gloves stops the knurled bar cutting into the palms of the hands. Also, as I have fairly large hands, the gloves effectively increase the circumference of the bar enabling me to exert a much stronger grip.

A tight closed grip is essential when the weight gets heavy, and not just for safety reasons. Psychologically it helps to really take hold of the bar with a strong grip rather than just letting it rest in your hands. You must feel to be in control of the bar - not the other way round. As one of my lifting partners always shouts to me just before I attempt a heavy lift - "come on now - take it strong!" He means grab it with a killer grip as you lift it off the pins. Mentally establish your dominance over the bar. Establish who is in charge. I find gloves definitely assist with my 'killer' grip.

If this is a day I want to give my muscles a real blast - a solid growth workout - I will now add 50lbs to the bar so my fourth set will look like this:

Olympic Bar	= 45lbs
Plus 2 x 45lb Plates	= 90lbs
Plus 2 x 25lb Plates	= 50lbs
Total Weight	= 185lbs

I will perform 6 reps of this fourth set, rest - then repeat, rest - then repeat again for a sixth set. It does not matter if I do not complete the full 6 reps on the fifth and sixth sets. I just lift to failure on these sets - which can of course mean that sometimes I will exceed the 6 reps. Remember lifting to failure means you carry on lifting, in each individual set, until you cannot complete another rep, thereby ensuring ***all*** the muscles fibres have been recruited.

For my seventh and final set I will then reduce the weight back down to just the bar and the 45 pound plates as follows:

Olympic Bar	= 45lbs
Plus 2 x 45lb Plates	= 90lbs
Total Weight	= 135lbs

I will perform 15 reps of this 'cool down' set which will then complete the bench press workout.

EXAMPLE 2

On another day my object may be to raise the threshold a bit in which case my workout will vary from the first example. The first 3 warm up sets will again remain the same but for my fourth set I will load an extra 15lbs to each end of the bar so it will look like this:

Olympic Bar	= 45lbs
Plus 2 x 45lb Plates	= 90lbs
Plus 2 x 10lb Plates	= 20lbs
Plus 2 x 5lb Plates	= 10lbs
Total Weight	= 165lbs

This is some 20 pounds lighter than my fourth set in the previous example but I am now going to complete 8 reps instead of 6. A real wake up call to my muscles to prime them for my fifth set where the weight will increase to 205 pounds by loading the bar as follows:

Olympic Bar	= 45lbs
Plus 2 x 45lb Plates	= 90lbs
Plus 2 x 35lb Plates	= 70lbs
Total Weight	= 205lbs

At this new weight I will attempt 5, 6 or 7 reps but always lift to failure to ensure overload. I will rest and then pyramid down to a total weight of 135 pounds for my sixth and final set - exactly as in the first example.

EXAMPLE 3

The third example of one of my bench press workouts is not so typical in that I would only attempt it every 10 to 12 weeks or so. It is purely an effort to establish, or improve upon, my 1RM rather than a proper workout.

A 1RM you will recall is the absolute maximum weight that can be lifted for just one repetition, with proper form, but no more (i.e. the weight is so heavy that a second repetition cannot be completed without assistance from a spotter).

It is not essential for the purposes of this book, and many people train successfully over the years, gaining large amounts of LBM in the process, without ever knowing or even wanting to know, their 1RM. All the 18 major benefits of strength will flow to you if you workout conscientiously as I have already described in examples 1 and 2. There is absolutely no requirement to try and establish a 1RM.

Having said that I have this irresistible curiosity to find out just how much weight I can actually lift. On a practical level a single figure target is much easier to remember than various numbers and combinations of sets and repetitions. Exceeding that target every couple of months or so is really exhilarating and will keep you motivated like nothing else will.

The 1RM on the bench press is probably the most universally understood bench mark of strength and can be meaningful even to those who do not workout at all. Whereas announcing to the world that you have just completed "3 sets of 10 reps of lying overhead dumbbell triceps extensions at 45 pounds" will just draw a blank stare - or maybe a suggestion that you should go and lie down for a while in a darkened room.

I repeat, this workout is absolutely optional, but if like me you feel inspired to find the limits of your strength the following example of my attempt on a new 1RM may be helpful. This particular example is one I attempted on 31st October 2005 just after turning 65 years of age.

Firstly, and as always, I completed the first 3 warm up sets exactly as in the previous two examples. I then rested for longer than normal - say 5 minutes - before proceeding with the next set for which I added the 25 pound plates to the bar. So the fourth set looked like this:

Olympic Bar	= 45lbs
Plus 2 x 45lb Plates	= 90lbs
Plus 2 x 25lb Plates	= 50lbs
Total Weight	= 185lbs

Exactly the same loading as the fourth set in my very first example, but this time I stopped after just 3 fairly quick reps. Again I rested for longer than usual - maybe up to 8 minutes this time.

Remember, this is not a normal strength building workout. My sole objective throughout this workout is to prepare my body for an attempt on a new or existing 1RM. I will therefore rest until I feel fully recovered, the only proviso being that I do not let my body cool down. I am also spinning out the time a bit to let my adrenaline fully kick in.

I then replaced the 25 pound plates with the 35 pound ones so the set up for the fifth set was as follows:

Olympic Bar	= 45lbs
Plus 2 x 45lb Plates	= 90lbs
Plus 2 x 35lb Plates	= 70lbs
Total Weight	= 205lbs

being exactly the same set up as the fifth set in my second example workout - but this time I only completed 2 reps in quick succession and absolutely no more. Again I rested for 5-8 minutes, probably doing a few reps on the cable machine at very light weights to keep my rotator cuff muscles warm. I then loaded 'the plates' so my sixth set looked like this:

Olympic Bar	= 45lbs
Plus 2 x 45lb Plates	= 90lbs
Plus 2 x 45lb Plates	= 90lbs
Total Weight	= 225lbs

I completed just 1 single rep at this weight, and no more - the last preparation set before I 'went for it'. My muscles were now as primed as they were ever going to be for an attempt on a new record. That last heavy rep was the final primer. I find it essential to lift a heavy weight in order to get the adrenaline flowing fully, but at the same time to perform the minimum number of reps in order to conserve energy for that final all out effort on a new personal best.

It is at this point that you need to be having a good day - feeling really strong - because from now on it is like shooting in the dark. Everything I have done up until now I have already done before. Now I have to guess what is the optimum amount of weight to load onto the bar for an attempt at a new personal best. How much extra weight should I load?

My advice is this: always err on the conservative side as it is quite depressing to fail at your first attempt - and at this point in time (you have already completed 6 preparation sets remember), and at this weight, you will not have the strength left for a second attempt. It is far better to load a weight at which you have a good chance of success because you will be really exhilarated at establishing your new 1RM.

As a start I would suggest loading the minimum increase that can be loaded, which is 5lbs (2 x 'the biscuits' which you will recall are the smallest plates and weigh 2.5 pounds each), to whatever weight you lifted for your previous 1RM.

If you feel you may have had a little left in the tank - no problem. That will help you decide on your next target. Far better to feel you may have been able to lift a little more than to fail. Increase the weight in small steps and bear in mind that when you attempt a new 1RM you are lifting at the absolute limit of your body's capacity. That is why it is so important to be feeling really good. Feeling really strong and psyched up at the end of that sixth and final set before entering uncharted waters.

If you have any doubts at all at this point just reduce the weight a little and complete a normal workout. Leave the new 1RM attempt for another day. It is just not worth attempting it unless you are feeling 110%.

If you are fairly new to lifting you will be amazed at the variation in your personal best between a 'good' and an 'off' day. In my case it can be as much as 25 to 30 pounds! So I repeat, never attempt a new 1RM unless you are feeling 110%.

That particular Monday afternoon of the 31st October 2005, I was feeling strong. Feedback from my spotter was good. He told me that I had made that final preparation rep at 225 pounds look easy. I was feeling energetic, warm and psyched up.

It was at that point, and only at that point, that I finally decided to try and establish a new 1RM. It was also comparatively easy for me, on that particular day, to decide what to shoot for as I had already lifted 230 pounds on a couple of previous occasions.

Accordingly I loaded the 5 pound plates giving a total weight of 235 pounds as follows:

Olympic Bar	= 45lbs
Plus 2 x 45lb Plates	= 90lbs
Plus 2 x 45lb Plates	= 90lbs
Plus 2 x 5lb Plates	= 10lbs
Total Weight	= 235lbs

This weight was now 5 pounds more than my previous 1RM (and would therefore be a new personal best for me) and 10 pounds more than the final preparation rep I had just completed. That may not sound much of an increase but when you are at the limit of your strength every extra pound feels like an extra ton.

Another reason I decided to shoot for 235 pounds was that it was the nice round figure of exactly 50 pounds more than my bodyweight, which on that particular day was 185 pounds. Without the experience I have now gained, and in a more reckless mood, I might have shot for 240 pounds - but had I failed I would have wasted all the preparation and been very, very disappointed.

There is no second chance - at least not on the same day, or possibly the same week allowing for recovery time. Once you fail on a big lift your strength vanishes - just as if a tap has been turned off. If I had attempted, and failed, at 240 pounds there is no way I could then have succeeded at the lower weight of 235 pounds.

In the event I lay down on the bench - feet as always planted firmly on the floor - grabbed the bar tightly and lifted it off the pins to lockout. I paused briefly and then lowered it slowly to my chest before pressing it back up to lockout position - thus successfully completing my new 1RM of 235 pounds and experiencing a feeling of total exhilaration. I had just lifted more weight than I had ever done in my life, and at the age of 65 to boot.

The key to success in bench pressing a heavy weight is to bring it down slowly. If you let gravity help bring the weight down (at its preferred acceleration of 32ft per second per second) the momentum will be such that you will never turn it around and press it back up again. You must always be in control of the bar, bringing it down both slowly, under control and without deviating from your normal movement. Once the bar moves out of line, either forwards or backwards, with a heavy weight on board, it is almost impossible to press it back up.

One further point before leaving this chapter on sets and repetitions is the question of getting assistance with lift off. That is having your spotter help you lift the bar off the pins to lockout - prior to starting the bench press.

There is no question that the initial lift off from the pins can consume a lot of energy when the weight is really heavy. After all the bar is slightly behind your head for the initial lift off.

However, I believe the psychological advantage may be lost to some extent if your spotter helps you lift the bar off the pins. You are not completely in control from the very beginning. You are not “taking it strong”. Others feel that any help is appreciated. The jury is split pretty well down the middle on this one and you will have to discover which way works best for you.

Finally, it has been pointed out to me that my emphasis on continually increasing the 1RM may be more appropriate to power lifters, rather than my stated aim of helping anyone to rollback 20 years through strength training. Absolutely not so. My sole aim is to demonstrate how anyone can reap the 18 benefits of increased muscle mass. Nothing is going to increase your muscle mass faster than continually increasing the amount you can lift.

Increasing the ***maximum*** amount you can lift from time to time adds a bit of fun to the process and, in my view, makes goal setting extremely simple because you are unlikely to ever forget this figure.

Chapter 25

Balanced Training

Here we are concerned with training all body parts uniformly, rather than the balance between training days and rest periods which is covered in the following chapter on recovery.

Nature does not seem to like unbalanced training and if you train one muscle excessively, while ignoring its counterpart, growth will be limited. For example, intensive and isolated training of the biceps, while ignoring the triceps, will result in an unbalanced arm and a limit to any long-term development. As the biceps contracts the triceps extends, and vice versa, and both muscles should be trained to the same extent, although not necessarily in the same workout.

As mentioned earlier, always start workouts with the major body exercises before going on to isolate specific muscles. Therefore on days you are training the upper body, start with the bench press, using either dumbbells or the Olympic bar. I almost always follow this with a triceps workout since these muscles have anyway been incorporated in the bench press to a greater or lesser extent, and are now fully warmed up.

The extent to which the triceps become involved in the bench press is governed by the width of the gip on the bar. The narrower the grip the more strain is applied to the triceps. Try a few presses (with a lighter weight) with your hands just 10 inches apart and your elbows pointing more forward and you will be performing an excellent triceps exercise. Whatever the grip on the bar may be, the biceps do not become involved at all in the bench press.

Continuing with an upper body workout I would then move onto the shoulders and then possibly the biceps. However, in practice I tend to train the biceps in the same workouts as I train the back. Rather like the triceps in the case of the bench press, the biceps will become involved to a greater or lesser extent in most back exercises and will likewise be suitably warmed up. How you constitute your workouts is a matter of personal choice but whatever your schedule is, if you train your triceps to failure once a week then you should apply the same intensity to the biceps.

Balance does not only apply to reciprocating pairs of muscles but also to body parts. So if you train the upper body intensely you should train the lower body to the same extent. If you exercise your front i.e. abdomen and chest through the bench press the same intensity should be applied to the development of your back muscles. In fact a strong back will benefit your bench press by providing a wide and stable base from which to press. More than this it will help you to avoid a shoulder injury such as the one I suffered several years ago.

Around my mid fifties I was really getting into the bench press - almost to the exclusion of everything else, including stretching which I never bothered with. At the time I had no knowledge of balanced training and just concentrated on the bench press - with disastrous results that kept me off the gym for a full 3 months.

What had happened was that my pectoral muscles had grown so strong and condensed (I was not aware of the importance of after workout stretching at the time) that they were pulling my shoulders forward. My under trained, and comparatively weak, back muscles were unable to restore the balance. It reached the point that when, as my physiotherapist at the time pointed out, I lay flat on my back my shoulders were about 4" off the couch.

Additionally, and as a direct result of this unbalanced training, the ligament which attaches the major pectoral muscles to the shoulder had become strained and inflamed and extremely painful when under any sort of pressure. Complete rest of this muscle was the order of the day so bench pressing was out - and stretching and back exercises were in until equilibrium had once again been re-established.

That said, balance is a matter of common sense and does not have to be taken to extremes. For example I exercise my upper arms extensively but not specifically my lower arms. This is because the forearms cannot but help being worked out by default during the course of most other exercises. Just picking up a pair of 100 pound dumbbells in preparation for some shoulder shrugs will work the forearms and wrists, and they will continue to be worked during the whole shoulder shrug exercise.

In fact just wandering around the gym with a 100 pound dumbbell in each hand will give the wrists and forearms a good workout. Try just such a wander for just 2 minutes or so and you will see exactly what I mean. My forearm size has certainly increased over the years despite no specific exercises for those particular muscles.

My training is not of course designed for someone wishing to enter a body building competition but purely to ensure that he/she continues to reap the benefits of all round strength, and I cannot overstress this point. If your objective is the truly immaculate body then each and every muscle must be targeted individually.

The sole aim of this book, however, is to enable you to develop enough lean body mass in order to reap the 18 benefits of increased strength for the rest of your life - nothing more. The next chapter deals with the all important issue of recovery - or the balance between days working out and rest days. All important because without proper recovery there will be no muscle growth at all.

Chapter 26

Recovery

Unless stress is applied to a muscle there will be no muscle growth whatsoever, as I hope I have demonstrated sufficiently in the preceding chapters. Stimulation in the form of stress is the number one essential ingredient for any increase in muscle mass.

However, recovery is a very, very close second. Without proper recovery any stress applied to a muscle will be a waste of time and effort as muscle growth cannot start until recovery is complete.

I mentioned earlier that when you exercise a muscle with heavy weights you are to all intents and purposes damaging it slightly. You are causing slight tears in the muscle fibres so that they can grow back stronger. And they certainly will. This is a natural body process that you don't even have to think about. All you have to do is to let the process happen. Simply let the repair and growth take place before subjecting that specific muscle to any further stress. This happens completely naturally and subconsciously and most recovery probably occurs while you are asleep.

So far very logical and just common sense. Break down the muscle fibres, let them recover, let them grow back bigger. Just allow this process to complete before repeating the cycle. Follow this formula and you virtually guarantee constantly increasing muscle mass.

The 64,000 dollar question, surrounded by controversy, is .just how long does this recovery process take? Well I can promise you this - the recovery process takes a lot longer than is generally thought. What I recommend below is based on trial and error over the last fifteen years - and I am the living proof as to how someone, at least someone in their fifties, can both continually and successfully increase muscle mass.

The biggest setback you are likely to experience in your quest for greater LBM is overtraining. At some point you will probably suffer from what has become known as Over Training Syndrome or OTS for short. This does ***not*** mean that you are training too hard or for too long. It does ***not*** mean that the weights are too heavy. What it ***does*** mean is that you are training too much, in that the intervals or recovery periods between workouts are too short.

It is vital not to confuse overload with overtraining. Overload is nature's way to boost performance through muscle growth, triggered as we have seen by the mobilisation of all the various muscle fibres through the use of heavy weights.

Overtraining means not allowing sufficient time for recovery and growth to take place before subjecting the muscles to further stress. Overload is to be encouraged. Overtraining, on the other hand, will result in 'plateauing' at best and injury at worst. This rather awkward word 'plateauing' simply means you have reached a plateau, where no further progress seems possible. However hard you try you simply can't manage any increase in the amount of weight being attempted.

In the extremely unlikely event that you have reached your absolute maximum physical potential you will suffer from plateauing. However 99 times out of 100 if you suffer from plateauing it is as a direct result of overtraining. You are suffering from OTS. During my years of trial and error I have over trained and suffered both plateauing and accidents as a result. The recommendations which follow will enable you to avoid both of these conditions.

I first became aware of plateauing in my mid fifties when I could not achieve any increase in the weight I was bench pressing. I am not talking here about a one off bad day which is quite normal and will happen to everyone from time to time.

Week in, week out, the weight I was able to lift remained stubbornly the same. In my frustration I increased my workout schedule from about 2 times a week to 3 or more. To my horror the amount of weight I was able to bench press actually started to go down.

Of course with hindsight it is easy to see the reason why. By increasing my schedule I was not allowing enough time for any proper recovery - let alone muscle growth. I was exercising my muscles when they were still partly damaged and torn down from the previous workout. My muscles were accordingly a bit weaker after that than at the start of the previous workout. Hardly surprising, therefore, that the amount of weight I was able to lift was actually reducing.

Back then I was still seduced by the ridiculous gym myth that you must workout Mondays, Wednesdays and Fridays in order to achieve any success. I promise you that schedule is a sure recipe for disaster. In my case the disaster finally occurred in the form of a torn ligament - the one that attaches the pectoral muscle to the shoulder - which resulted in a 3 month layoff and many sessions with the physiotherapist. The day of my accident (the day the ligament tore) is described in Chapters 25 and 28 because it also relates directly to both balanced training and safe lifting.

Having to take 3 months off when you are trying to increase your bench press is really frustrating and disappointing. So much hard work gone to waste. The knowledge that the 'accident' was caused purely by self inflicted ignorant training methods, rather than an unpredictable and unavoidable third party event, like the roof falling in, does not help much either.

On reflection, how much better to take an extra day or two off a week rather than an enforced layoff of 3 months. However, every cloud, I believe, really does have a silver lining, and in my case the 3 month layoff inspired me to research the optimum training frequency. Those researches, in conjunction with the ensuing ten years of practical experience, have enabled me to establish the ideal workout schedule that will ensure continuing progress.

I started by trying to establish how much time someone could take off resistance training before any measurable decrease in muscle strength occurred. I was already fully aware of the maxim 'if you don't use it you will lose it' - but don't use it for how long precisely? The answer to this will vary depending on the sport, exercise, activity and type of training being undertaken.

The results of my research, and my following recommendations, apply ***only*** to resistance training where the muscles are subjected to overload - as defined in Chapter 23. Most aerobic activity can be undertaken on an almost daily basis with no side affects. Many sports require less recovery time than heavy resistance training. Top tennis players for example would be ill advised to consistently take off the number of recovery days I suggest. In addition to applying only to resistance training, my suggestions are ***only*** applicable to fit individuals who have been following a weight training programme for 6 months or more.

During the first three months of weight training, in order to increase LBM, progress is usually quite dramatic - and this initial three month spurt seems to apply regardless of the age at which you start. During this period recovery times can, in practice, be decided by how your body feels. That will be dictated by the speed of elimination of the lactic acid which is what causes stiffness. If you find all stiffness gone after 3 days then it is probably safe to hit the weights again. But as your muscles get larger recovery times must get longer if you wish that initial growth to continue on a consistent basis.

Finally, my personal experience is only based on the last 15 years, as I did not take up resistance training until I had just turned 50. However, my researches and observations indicate that you need to increase your recovery periods as you progress (with the proviso that you have consistently trained to failure for at least six months) ***regardless*** of the age at which you start. Thus two individuals, who have followed the same intensive resistance programme for say, two years, will need to increase their recovery periods by the same identical amounts - despite the fact that one is aged 29 and the other 47.

Recovery time, I believe, is dictated more by increase in muscle mass than by increase in age. I should mention here that the whole of this chapter is concerned with the correct number of recovery days between workouts in order to sustain continuing muscle growth. I am ***not*** concerned here with recovery, or resting times, between the individual sets of an exercise. Those resting periods, which may vary from one up to say ten minutes, are to a large extent dictated by overall fitness levels - as opposed to just strength - and may well indeed lengthen with age. That is not my concern here.

It is worth repeating: my ***sole*** objective was to establish the ideal workout schedule that would ensure the maximum muscle growth, on a continuing basis, through resistance training. The 'ideal workout schedule' is one where the recovery period is restricted to sufficient days to allow full repair of muscle fibres and total completion of new muscle growth - and no more.

It is ideal because it is also the most efficient in that the next workout follows on as soon as possible. However, there is no harm in giving your body a further day's holiday from time to time. In fact when unforeseen appointments or events crop up on a scheduled training day my advice is always to postpone the workout, rather than to bring it forward by a day. It is just not worth the risk of subjecting muscles to further stress before any new growth has fully completed.

To recap, my starting point therefore was to establish how much time someone could take off resistance training before any measurable decrease in muscle strength occurred. In other words to establish the absolute maximum parameter for recovery. My experience, and the consensus of many experienced trainers, is that 14 days without any resistance training will result in negligible loss of strength. Beyond 14 days reduction in peak strength may start to become significant. So 14 days becomes my absolute maximum parameter. This is quite a convenient number as it happens to fit in with a lot of holiday schedules. A happy coincidence.

My second step was to try and establish the absolute minimum parameter. Again with the same proviso: applicable only to fit individuals who have been following a weight training programme for 6 months or more.

The evidence here was often based more on what doesn't work rather than on what does - ie the complete lack of progress observed in many individuals over the years who insisted on working out every other day. Such individuals may be fitter but they were certainly not achieving their desired goal of increasing LBM. It was almost as if the working out had become an end in itself rather than a means to reap all the benefits of increased strength. Working out every other day can never work because the body has simply not had the time to recover.

I use the word body on purpose because it is not just the muscles that have to recover. The eliminatory organs such as the liver and kidneys will be working overtime during the next 24 hours following a heavy workout expelling the acidic build up caused directly by that workout.

The organs don't care that you may be resting the pectoral muscles and working the legs instead - they still have to get rid of the impurities no matter which body part caused the build up in the first place. Judging purely from the absence of stiffness, this recovery process can take anything from 1 to 4 days - giving me an absolute minimum of 2 days required for recovery. Muscle growth probably takes longer than recovery although I can only prove this through my own experience (see below). However, assuming growth only requires the same amount of time as recovery; this still gives another minimum period of two days for growth - or 4 days in all.

So 4 is my absolute minimum parameter - the minimum number of rest days that must be allowed between intensive workouts of the ***same*** body part in order to achieve consistent increase in muscle mass. So, for example, and using this minimum recovery period, if I bench press to failure on a Saturday I must allow at least 4 days rest before bench pressing again on the following Thursday - or I will risk sabotaging muscle growth.

At this point I have now established a **minimum** parameter of 4 days rest, to enable recovery and growth to take place, and a **maximum** parameter of 14 days rest. Any number of days rest taken in between those figures of 4 and 14 will almost certainly result in long term muscle growth - but not in a very efficient manner.

My aim, remember, was to establish the optimum recovery period, which I define as being *the **least** number of rest days required between working out the same body part to failure that will allow the maximum, consistent increase in muscle mass of that body part.* That is a number of days that falls somewhere between 4 and 14.

The foregoing is somewhat theoretical and what really matters is what works best in practice. I am fortunate to have had 15 years of such practice, and one of the most valuable discoveries I have made has nothing to do with sets, repetitions, weights, training techniques or sports nutrition. It has to do with recovery - and it is this: 4 days rest is **not** sufficient to allow maximum muscle growth. Some growth will occur, especially in the first few months, and possibly in the first few years, of resistance training, but not the maximum possible. As the muscles get larger the more time they need for recovery if continuing growth (as opposed to just maintenance) is the aim. In order to achieve ongoing muscle growth a full 6 days rest between workouts of the same body part is needed. Longer rest intervals of say 8 or 9 days will do absolutely no harm but will probably not result in any further growth either.

In earlier chapters I have discussed the 1 rep maximum lift or 1RM. I stress again that attempting a 1RM is not a requirement of resistance training in order to increase LBM. You will obtain all the benefits of strength training without ever establishing your own 1RM. Having said that, I personally find it both exciting and motivating to try and establish a new 1RM from time to time.

On the occasions that I have both attempted **and** succeeded in increasing my 1RM on **consecutive** workouts the recovery period has invariably been 6 or 7 days. Longer or shorter intervals have always resulted in failure. This is the real practical proof that gives me the optimum recovery period. This is not theory.

When you attempt a new 1RM you are attempting to lift more weight than you have ever done in your life. A new pinnacle. To further increase that pinnacle on a **consecutive** workout requires the optimum recovery period.

Thus through trial and error I have established the full body workout schedule that incorporates the optimum recovery periods. It would be tidy and convenient if it covered exactly a week but that does not allow quite enough time. My schedule requires 8 days for full body training. How the training sessions are allocated between body parts is a matter of personal preference. A lot of people simply train the upper body on one day and the lower body on another, and there is nothing wrong with that.

As mentioned earlier I prefer to workout the biceps following major back exercises, and the triceps following the bench press, as both muscles have been involved to some extent in the major exercises and consequently are already warmed up.

My workouts are therefore allocated as follows:

Workout A 'The Presses' being the bench press, triceps press and various shoulder presses.

Workout B 'LABB' standing for legs, abdomen, back and biceps

As stated above my optimum recovery period is 6 or 7 days. Choosing 7 days recovery allows an identical number of days off between workouts which is easier to remember. My ideal schedule is therefore as follows:

Day 1	Monday	**Workout A**
Day 2	Tuesday	rest day
Day 3	Wednesday	rest day
Day 4	Thursday	rest day
Day 5	Friday	**Workout B**
Day 6	Saturday	rest day
Day 7	Sunday	rest day
Day 8	Monday	rest day
Day 9	Tuesday	**Workout A**

This schedule allows the full 7 days rest between working out the ***same*** body part, while requiring only 2 trips to the gym a week.

In week 1 (as above) workout days are Monday and Friday. In week 2 workout days will be Tuesday and Saturday - and so on. After a couple of months you will have visited the gym at least once on every day of the week and thus had the opportunity to meet everyone there. Much more interesting I think than a same day cycle. Follow a similar schedule and you can rest assured that you are allowing your body sufficient time for full recovery and maximum growth.

Time and time again I come across individuals who cannot understand why muscle growth has slowed, or more usually stopped altogether - the so called plateauing syndrome - despite intensified workouts.

Well, it is just because of those intensified workouts, and the perceived solution of working out even more often just makes the problem get worse. The correct solution is to allow time for proper recovery. If you ever find yourself in a plateauing situation my advice is to avoid the gym completely for a full two weeks. Rest, relax and eat well and you will be pleasantly surprised at your results when you return. Good nutrition, the sixth ingredient of my optimal routine, covered next, can certainly enhance that muscle growth.

Chapter 27

Nutrition

As we have seen in Chapter 2 'Reduce Body Fat and Increase Lean Body Mass' exercising at a low intensity is fuelled mostly by fat. As the intensity increases (as in lifting heavy weights) the body switches to glycogen for fuel, requiring ample supplies of carbohydrates. So carbohydrates are essential to supply the energy to exercise the muscle. Protein is equally essential to help the muscle recover, rebuild and sustain further growth after exercising.

The third vital nutrient required for a healthy body is fat – but the right fat. The inclusion of these three nutrients, (carbohydrate, protein and fat) in any eating plan is universally accepted. The arguments start over the relative quantities of each nutrient. These range from the 'Atkins' type diet at the one extreme – high protein and fat content combined with low carbs – to the very low fat, high carbs diet at the other extreme.

Neither of these extremes will assist your strength training but will almost certainly sabotage your efforts. To confuse the issue even further it is practically impossible to track the amount of fat you consume, short of turning your kitchen into a laboratory. The truth (as always it seems) lies somewhere in the middle.

Over the last 15 years I have experimented with increasing the amount of protein in my diet (at the expense of carbohydrate rather than fat) with absolutely no noticeable difference in muscle gain. To me this certainly endorses the current consensus view that increasing protein intake in order to build extra muscle is a waste of time. The fact that the hunks and strongmen you may see on TV do consume huge amounts of protein is irrelevant - because it is their very intense workouts that build their muscles, and not all that extra protein.

To quote the pretty successful body builder Arnold Schwarzenegger "...more than 2 grams of protein for every kilogram of bodyweight is unnecessary". That is a lot less than you might think - amounting to just 160 grams for a man weighing 80 kilograms. I think you will agree that 160 grams would not be considered an overly large sized steak. In fact some people would consider it to be quite a small steak. Nevertheless, I am entirely convinced that it is unnecessary to increase protein intake beyond this amount (2 grams of protein for every kilogram of bodyweight) in order to build new muscle.

As you will see by the end of this chapter my diet has altered little, in volume, over the years (experimentation apart) since I picked up my first dumbbell aged 50. My biceps, however, have probably increased by 4 inches - and thanks to lifting to failure, rather than any increase in protein intake. Having that bigger steak will certainly not harm you, but neither will it give you any additional benefit in terms of muscle growth.

So my recommendation regarding protein intake is to improve the quality rather than the quantity. By quality I also mean protein that is most easily absorbed by the body. Lean meat, fish, eggs and, by far and away at the top of the list, whey protein powder. Whey protein is most easily used by the body, and also the most easily prepared and consumed, particularly in sports shakes (more on whey protein later).

Of course some of that steak will not be protein but fat - saturated fat in fact. How much fat will depend on the particular animal concerned (wild, not farmed, venison will have much less fat than beef) as well as the specific cut of meat and the quality. The amount of fat can vary from 5% - 35% but what is certain is that you will never know for sure unless, as mentioned earlier, you turn your kitchen into a laboratory.

Any diet that advises you to consume fixed percentages of the three nutrients in the following proportions of, say, carbohydrate 40%, protein 30% and fat 30% is well meaning but is being totally impracticable. The only ingredients you can measure with any hope of accuracy are a very small number of carbohydrate nutrients and pure fats like, say, 5 grams of olive oil. Fancy including an avocado with your diet lunch? Well you have really got problems because every avocado contains protein, fat ***and*** carbohydrate in varying but significant proportions, depending on a multitude of factors which you cannot possibly determine.

Over the years I have found it quite unnecessary to count calories or measure ingredients whether by percentage or by weight. Provided you eat a healthy diet (as defined below) your body will automatically control how much you consume by regulating your hunger. Measuring and counting ingredients and calories is both impractical and cannot anyway be accurate.

A few simple rules and plenty of common sense are all that are required to eat in the healthiest possible manner. I think the majority of people reading this far will already be eating a fairly healthy diet, so I will limit this chapter on nutrition to a few eating tips and strategies which I have found can enhance muscle growth in conjunction with resistance training. Firstly my definition of a healthy diet.

I mentioned in the introduction to this book that I had found strength to be a totally natural attribute of a healthy body, because I believed that strength had been, for hundreds of thousands of years, an essential ingredient to survival.

Likewise, our bodies have evolved over the same many millennia from the way we ate. The comparatively recent arrival of civilisation, and consequent crop cultivation and animal husbandry, has dramatically altered our eating habits - and in the blink of an eye, as it were, in terms of evolution. Our stomachs have evolved over millions of years, and in my view will need many millions more to learn to absorb man made molecules of 'food' such as, for example, those found in margarine and other substances containing hydrogenated fats or trans fatty acids.

These fats are not found in nature. Hydrogenated fats are the result of complex chemical processes involving high temperatures, bleaching, distillation and the addition of preservatives, all of which are designed to keep oils (that would otherwise be liquid) solid at room temperature. These processes increase shelf-life (by preventing the oil from becoming rancid), ease of handling and usability and, together with cheaper ingredients than their natural counterparts, boost profitability for manufacturers. They are the ultimate processed 'food'. Wherever you see the words 'hydrogenated' or 'partially hydrogenated' on the contents label of a product, put it back on the shelf.

So the number one rule in my definition of a healthy diet is this: avoid ***all*** processed food as much as possible - and avoid hydrogenated fats (trans fatty acids) like the plague. They will probably kill you. A diet of processed food is more than likely the root cause of every modern disease and cancer.

I am old enough to remember a government minister appearing on TV in the early sixties in order to reassure us all that smoking was not in fact harmful. I recall, a few years later, advertisements depicting, a presumably rather simple, blonde announcing to her friend that she could not tell the difference between margarine and butter. Well, time changes everything, and I believe that the day is not far off when margarine will be subject to the same health warnings that cigarettes are now - “MARGARINE KILLS”. [Unsalted butter, although a saturated fat, has in fact been subjected to the absolute minimum of processing - just churning - and is at least full of naturally formed nutrients].

It is interesting to note that one of America’s largest and more enlightened coffee and snack retailers - Starbucks - is already withdrawing products made with hydrogenated fats from its counters in many US outlets.

New York has become the first American city to introduce a program of banning artificial ‘trans fats’ including partially hydrogenated vegetable oils, from restaurants and other eateries. I believe other cities, and countries, will follow suite as more people become aware of the hidden dangers in many fats, and even more importantly, the damage ***processing*** can do to otherwise healthy fats and oils.

That is why my main rule to healthy nutrition is to avoid ***all*** processing as much as possible. Even cooking is a process - so the more raw fruit and vegetables you can eat the better. Cooking or applying high heat to many vegetable oils will cause them to become unstable. Some vegetable oils will oxidise very quickly once opened or exposed to strong light.

Using a cooking oil that is simply labelled ‘vegetable oil’ or even ‘pure vegetable oil’ may at first sight appear to be a healthy option but it is almost guaranteed to be made from oils that have been extracted by chemical means at high temperatures. Furthermore, it is almost as certainly guaranteed to be a blend high in poly-unsaturated fats such as those found in safflower, corn, sunflower and soybean vegetable oils.

It is generally believed that all unsaturated fats are healthy but this is not the case. Poly-unsaturated fats are bad for your health when consumed in excessive amounts. They should be avoided. They do not have any redeeming health benefits but are widely used by food manufacturers because they are ***cheap***.

The healthy option is to use oils that have been extracted solely by pressing (mechanical means) rather than by the application of heat (chemical means). Such oils are usually labelled 'cold pressed'.

The king of the lot is Extra Virgin Olive Oil for the simple reason that it can stand reasonably high temperatures and so is ideal for cooking. There are several other beneficial, cold pressed oils widely available now such as walnut, avocado and flaxseed to name a few but these oils should only be used as cold dressings - and ***never*** heated. To keep life simple I stick entirely to Extra Virgin Olive Oil for both cooking and salad dressings. This oil is always cold pressed and ideally should also be both unfiltered and unrefined. Olive oil, although monounsaturated (as opposed to polyunsaturated), is rich in Omega-6 fatty acids and you will still need to balance this with foods rich in Omega-3 fatty acids - such as oily fish, walnuts, avocados, flaxseeds and green leafy vegetables for example.[4]

Sticking to my number one rule of avoiding all processed food as much as possible also involves skipping refined sugar and salt.

Refining is a process - a process even more damaging than cooking can be. Chances are that if a substance is pure white it is refined. White sugar is the only food that provides no fibre, vitamins, minerals or other beneficial nutrients whatsoever. Refined sugar is not only completely useless nutritionally but positively damaging, breaking down into acid and playing havoc with the delicate balance of a variety of bodily processes - never mind rotting the teeth and gums! High consumption of sugar will actually interfere with the absorption of many other

---

[4] The subject of fats and oils is quite complex and well beyond the scope of this book. If you wish to investigate further I highly recommend "Fats that Heal, Fats that Kill" by Udo Erasmus, an internationally recognised authority on the subject.

vital nutrients such as manganese, thus nullifying the benefit of any of those expensive supplements you may be taking.

In Chapter 11 we saw how strength training actually improves you body's sensitivity to insulin, making just a little of this hormone go a long way. However, consuming foods high in refined sugar will sabotage this benefit by causing excess glucose in your blood, which triggers the release of insulin, which in turn will lower the glucose levels. So that the more sugary foods you consume the final result is a lowering of blood sugar! Surely a viscous circle to avoid at all costs.

Pure white (refined) salt is as equally damaging as white sugar. Salt (sodium chloride) is a wonderful preservative that played a vital role in the days before fridges and commercial freezing. It preserves by extracting water, and other liquids from whatever it touches.

Quite simply it dehydrates you, a fact used ruthlessly by the major brewing houses who ensure that any 'snacks' available at their licensed premises are highly salted. Thus the acidic packet of crisps, or salted toasted nuts, you just consumed has to be washed down by yet more acidic beer in order to quench the resultant thirst. A double whammy - and never mind the processed fat content of the crisps!

Many nutritionists consider salt to be the primary cause of high blood pressure which leads directly to increased risk of stroke, heart disease and kidney failure. Salt not only decreases the amount of calcium your body is able to absorb, but simultaneously increases the amount you excrete[5]. Another double whammy!

Eating a healthy diet and particularly avoiding processed foods as discussed above will ensure that your body is in the best possible condition to reap all of the benefits of strength training. However, there are 4 specific ways in which I have found that strength gains can be enhanced through small adjustments to an already healthy diet.

For the purposes of maximising muscle growth a low fat diet cannot be considered healthy as it lowers testosterone lev-

---

[5] Edith Hogan RD - American Dietetic Association (see Food Remedies p397)

els, whatever else it may or may not do. The 4 adjustments I recommend are as follows:-

1) Eat protein and carbohydrate together.

Foods rich in carbohydrates will affect the amount of insulin that your body secretes. When eaten alone they will cause blood sugar peaks and troughs which in turn will affect both your performance and your mood. If protein is consumed simultaneously it will slow down and steady the absorption of the carbohydrates, keeping insulin secretion on an even keel.

So when snacking always choose, say, half a wholemeal chicken sandwich over a sugared doughnut. If you follow my advice about processed food you should not be contemplating the sugared doughnut anyway! Also because protein takes longer to digest than carbohydrates you will feel fuller longer if you combine the two.

Eating highly sugared carbohydrate snacks on their own will reinforce the vicious circle in blood sugar levels mentioned earlier in this chapter, actually making you feel more hungry than you were before you started.

On days when I have a heavy afternoon workout ahead I often eat a bowlful of oat porridge for lunch, but I ***always*** add a scoopful (20 grams) of whey protein powder. I also usually add a tablespoon of ground flaxseed and sweeten the whole lot with a tablespoon of blackstrap molasses. When mixed it closely resembles the mash we used to feed the horses on race days in the stable where I worked as a student. This combination worked for the horses and it certainly works for me; energy from the oats, protein from the whey powder and fat (Omega 3 fatty acids in this case) from the flaxseeds.

In my experience, combining protein, carbohydrates and fats as much as possible whenever you eat will not only improve your workouts (and thus your results) but also diminish body fat retention.

The one exception to this rule is fruit. Always eat fruit raw and preferably on its own. Cooking fruit, and tomatoes, simply turns a naturally alkaline food into an acidic one. I also snack on dried fruit such as prunes, apricots, figs and dates but they all contain concentrated levels of sugar, albeit in the natural form of fructose, so should only be eaten in small quantities.

2) Have both a pre and post workout snack

You need protein to build muscles but you also need that protein to help your muscles recover and repair - and the sooner after a heavy workout the better. Immediately after strenuous resistance training your muscles will be primed for growth but that growth must be fuelled by both protein and carbohydrates. The carbohydrate will replenish glycogen levels and the protein will repair tissue. Both are essential in order to maximise muscle growth.

However, it is equally important to have a snack containing both carbohydrate and protein just before a heavy workout. This will not only keep your energy levels high during the workout but also the protein will ensure the availability of amino acids throughout the workout, thus avoiding any possible cannibalization of the muscles.

These pre and post workout snacks can be taken in many forms but the one most efficiently absorbed by the body is liquid - in the form of a sports or so called 'protein' shake. This is where whey protein really comes into its own.

Whey protein is the name for a collection of globular proteins that can be isolated from whey, a by-product of cheese manufactured from cow's milk. It is typically a mixture of beta-lactoglobulin (65%), alpha-lactalbumin (25%), and serum albumin (8%), which are soluble in their native forms. Whey has the highest Biological Value (BV) of any known protein and is digested rapidly thus allowing fast uptake of amino acids. Being in powder form it is the perfect protein to add to an otherwise carbohydrate sports drink.

There are literally hundreds of recipes for sports drinks widely available in magazines and on the Internet but the one I use is as follows. It is one of the easiest to prepare and nutritionally cannot be bettered as a workout snack. Simply put the following ingredients in a blender:

1 cup yoghurt
1 chopped banana
1 scoop whey protein powder (20 grams)

1 teaspoon honey

Add milk or soy milk as necessary to adjust the consistency

Blend all.

That's it. A simple classic. You can also add some ground flax-seed or any piece of fruit you have hanging around if desired. A couple of strawberries, half a pear etc. will add variety to the flavour.

I try and make double the quantity on workout days so that I can drink half just before I leave for the gym, and freeze the other half to take with me. In theory it should be melted and ready to drink by the time I finish my workout but in practice I usually have to spend a few minutes in the steam room de-frosting it. However, there are days when there is no time to prepare a shake, or the necessary ingredients are not to hand.

On occasions I have even forgotten to take the prepared shake from the freezer when leaving for the gym. In these instances the next best bet is a protein or sports bar. It should contain around 30% protein. Again, these are not always readily available in which case I have often resorted to buying a simple wholemeal chicken or ham and cheese sandwich. I eat one half immediately before and the other half immediately after my workout. Not ideal - but far, far better than being tempted by the hundreds of readily available snacks which are nothing but carbohydrates, sugar and, usually, hydrogenated fats. Without the protein the muscles cannot repair efficiently. Consuming a quality sports drink both pre and post workout will aid muscle repair and enhance muscle growth.

3) Eat frequently - about every 2½ hours

Eating frequently will keep blood sugar levels more constant throughout the day thus avoiding swings in mood and energy. Equally importantly the metabolism is kept fired up all day thus assisting with the reduction in body fat percentage as covered in Chapter 2. However, eating frequently does not mean eating more but eating the same amount spread over a greater number of meals.

Some sports nutritionists recommend eating as many as 6 meals a day, which I think will be impractical for most people.

My suggestion is that you stick to the 3 main meals, but cut the amounts by having just one course at each, and introduce two smaller meals around 11.00am and 4.00pm. These two smaller meals can take the form of snacks such as a sandwich or a packet of some dried fruit and nuts. In fact there is no reason why a sports or protein shake should be reserved for gym days. It is the perfect replacement or fill-in meal. Keeping your body fully fuelled will ensure you never run out of energy in the gym.

4) Drink plenty of water

Water is vital for every single bodily function and process and it is almost impossible to have too much of it. Most people are in fact walking around in a semi dehydrated state. The recommended daily quantity is usually given as being 8 glasses, which is pretty meaningless.

If you are undertaking strength training you need to be fully hydrated in order to assist muscle performance and growth. I would recommend 3 litres as being nearer the mark for daily intake - which may be 8 glasses, or it may indeed be 16, depending of course on the size of your glass.

Drink plenty of water before, during and after working out to ensure the maximum benefit and to assist the complex biological processes of recovery and repair that are taking place. I usually consume 1.5 litres while in the gym. Drinking water without resistance training will not of course make you one jot stronger - but drinking water as you train will definitely facilitate both your performance and your results.

These 4 adjustments to your otherwise healthy diet, made in conjunction with the strength training routines described in this book, will assist in maximising your Lean Body Mass and strength.

Finally, before leaving this chapter on nutrition, a quick word on supplementation. On page 13 I questioned the value of taking calcium supplements but would otherwise certainly recommend taking at least the vitamins C, E and the B group, which I consider to be the basics.

However, here I am talking about strength training supplements rather than vitamins. The one most widely used, debated and researched has to be creatine, a substance produced naturally by the body anyway.

There have been studies proving its effectiveness in improving many medical conditions[6], sporting performance and just about everything else - and there have been other studies showing it has little or no impact on muscle growth. However, none of the many studies have been able to show that creatine supplementation has any harmful side effects.

Creatine is advertised as being particularly effective in sports requiring sudden bursts of strength such as in resistance training. I have certainly experimented with it on and off over the last few years in an effort to improve my bench press but so far I cannot say that it has made any difference to my results. My intuition suggests that any difference in anyone else will be marginal at best. On the other hand those who use it regularly swear by it. Anyway it seems to be safe so my advice has to be to give it a try if you wish.

No supplementation, however, can replace proper nutrition. For muscles to grow it is essential to feed the body with healthy nutrients, and the simplest way to achieve that is to avoid all processed and refined foods whenever possible. Snack on a piece of fruit, for example, rather than on a piece of fruit cake. Beyond that, the 4 adjustments I suggest in this chapter should ensure that your diet is optimised for maximum muscle growth.

---

[6] See Life Extension magazine - March 2003 issue

Chapter 28

Safe Lifting, Correct Form & Technique

Lifting safely is vital if you want to be around long enough to enjoy all the benefits of this increased LBM. A lot of safe lifting is common sense - like having an able spotter in position if you are intending to bench press to failure - but a lot comes from correct form and lifting technique which are not always intuitive but have to be learnt, preferably via a live demonstration from your gym instructor.

Correct form not only ensures you are lifting safely but that you are also exercising any specific muscle/muscle group in the most efficient manner. There are many publications available illustrating every conceivable exercise and you will find links on my website www.williamfaro.com to my recommended ones.

However, nothing beats a live demonstration from a qualified instructor who can not only demonstrate the exercise but also then make sure you are performing it correctly - something it is often difficult to check for yourself even with the benefit of mirrors. In fact for all but the simplest exercises it is worth getting a colleague or instructor to cast a critical eye over your performance every few months or so. It is only too easy to lose correct form imperceptibly over the weeks. Here I am not talking about the correct form that simply isolates a particular muscle but the correct form that is essential for safe lifting.

An example of the former would be allowing the elbows to spread during a lying triceps EZ bar extension where the bar is lowered to just above the bridge of the nose. Strictly correct form stipulates that your elbows should be pointing forward. Letting them spread engages some support from other muscles so that the triceps are no longer strictly isolated and the exercise accordingly becomes easier. Not correct form, but still a very useful exercise and you will certainly benefit from it. The point is that in this instance deviating from correct form has no repercussions on safety - just on efficiency or specific targeting.

However, not observing correct form while performing squats; whether by not holding your stomach in tightly, or by not holding your shoulder blades together, will have possibly disastrous repercussions on your back. Both of these deviations from correct form can be difficult to check in a mirror especially when you are head on to it.

Another potentially dangerous tendency while performing squats is to let the knees move forward, rather than the seat move backward, as you lower your trunk. Again this is very difficult to check in a mirror from a head on view. However, an instructor watching you side on will immediately spot this tendency. My advice therefore has to be: by all means study the best illustrations of exercises (via my website for example) but ***always*** get a qualified instructor to demonstrate every exercise the first time you attempt it. This is now a mandatory requirement in most modern gyms anyway with suitable notices posted adjacent to each exercise machine. Equally importantly ***always*** get that instructor to then check your form as you in turn execute the exercise for the first time. Keep re-checking your form, at least from the perspective of safety, every few months.

Knowledge about the potential damage that certain exercises may have on the body is continually improving. Some exercises that were supported 10 years ago are now definitely discouraged - at least in enlightened gyms. The ones I am most concerned about involve the shoulder joint which is such a vital component in the bench press. Any upper body exercise where the shoulders are externally rotated, and the hands are behind the head, places the shoulder in the dislocation (unstable) position. It also places undue stress on the neck and increases the possibility of tendon strain.

Drawing on my personal experience I would not just discourage you from performing such exercises but suggest that if you do persist you are almost guaranteed to damage your shoulder joint at some point in time - just as I did.

Such exercises are definitely ***not*** safe. So never pull down (as in lat pull downs for example) or press up (as in the shoulder press) a bar behind your head. Always keep the bar in front of you. It is of course fine to hold the bar behind the neck when performing squats since no strain is placed on the shoulder joint.

I would also highly recommend that when bench pressing you only lower the bar, as a rule, to within 3 or 4 inches of your chest - and no lower. This again is to avoid the possibility of putting the shoulder in the dislocation position. Of course the larger your chest, and the more you arch your back, the less likelihood there is of this happening anyway.

Although the major shoulder muscles are not involved in the bench press to anything like the extent that the triceps and pectoral muscles are, the actual shoulder joint is of course bearing ***all*** of the weight. The massive amount of weight on the Olympic bar is ultimately connected to your body via the shoulder joints. This is why it is so important to take every possible precaution to protect the shoulders - particularly proper warming up as specifically discussed for the shoulders in Chapter 22.

Outside of competitive lifting there is no reason at all why the bar should touch the chest. It is the amount of weight that you are pressing, rather than the range of motion that will determine the increase in muscle mass. I say as a rule because I have no problem with, very occasionally, bouncing the bar off my chest. I hasten to add this is considered bad form by purists - but not on safety grounds. It is considered bad form because your muscles receive a brief respite during the bounce. So what? I find that when pressing weights close to my bodyweight with quick repetitions just touching my chest helps the rhythm and usually enables me to add another rep or two. Never try this technique with really heavy weights, or it definitely will become bad form on safety grounds, possibly cracking your sternum.

In Chapter 24 I referred to a shoulder injury I had sustained as a result of over training, and how the absence of stops on the bar saved me from a more serious accident. It may be helpful to examine what actually happened so you can avoid making the same mistakes.

For some weeks I had been suffering from what I now know to be Over Training Syndrome. At the time I had never heard of OTS and just assumed my lack of progress was due to not trying hard enough. Consequently I redoubled my efforts, visiting the gym 3 or 4 times a week. This was simply making a bad situation worse. I was unintentionally weakening my muscles by giving them no time for recovery, let alone growth. Also I was mistakenly 'working through' the pain in my right shoulder. A terrible mistake. Pain is nature's way of saying stop, or you will compound any damage. I am talking here about real pain in a joint - not just muscle stiffness or soreness which can usually be safely worked through.

My frustration was mounting as the amount of weight I was able to bench press was actually starting to decline! One day, in a desperate effort to halt this reverse, I loaded the bar with a weight I knew I had lifted six months earlier and, in a mood of defiance, lifted it off the pins to lockout. This was an unplanned lift and consequently I had no spotter - another terrible mistake. As soon as I started to lower the bar my right shoulder, already abused by OTS, just simply collapsed.

My right arm might as well as have been made of cotton wool for all the good it did in trying to halt the descent of the fully loaded Olympic bar, which consequently came racing down towards my right shoulder. My left arm was still supporting the other end of the bar just below lockout so that a split second before impact the bar was at an angle of about 45 degrees. Just as I felt my left arm also starting to collapse under the increased weight, there was a deafening crash as the plates on the right end slid off thc bar smashing onto the floor.

Relieved of some 80 pounds worth of plates the now empty right end of the bar shot back up into the air at the precise moment that my left arm finally gave way. Another 45 degree angle (but this time from the left side) and another deafening crash as all the plates on the left end of the bar slid onto the floor. People came running .... to find me sheepishly pressing a now empty bar back onto the pins. A very embarrassing situation but at least I was unharmed.

It is worth considering what could have happened if I had placed the so called safety stops at each end of the bar to stop the plates falling off. Following the collapse of my right arm the plates would have remained firmly in place so that when my left arm also collapsed I would have had a one inch thick bar now weighing some 200 pounds lying across my chest. Apart from crushing the breath out of me and cracking my ribs the bar, assisted by gravity, may well have rolled on down across my neck with possibly fatal consequences.

I made many mistakes that day and recount this episode purely in the hope that it may help you avoid similar ones. Of course the one lesson that this example is emphatically endorsing is ***always*** have a competent spotter when bench pressing free weights.

Finally a word on technique. A lot of technique is acquired naturally simply by gaining familiarity with the process involved. The body will learn at a subconscious level without too much specific input. However strong you may be to start with, bench pressing 150 pounds will always be easier the second or third time you attempt it.

Likewise the first day you decide to walk 3 miles before breakfast will always seem harder than the third time you try it. By the end of 2 weeks you will not even think about it.

I have often watched, and sometimes assisted, removal men moving heavy and awkward objects from one of my homes to the next. Even men of a very slight build, apparently physically weaker than me, handle loads with a dexterity and speed with which I just cannot compete. They of course do their job day in and day out and their bodies have evolved a technique that more than makes up for my possibly superior strength. In the gym this technique can be acquired fairly quickly. In my experience by the third attempt at a new exercise any feelings of being daunted will have been dispelled by the progress being achieved. This early improvement is due to naturally acquired technique rather than greater strength.

There is another aspect to technique which does require some specific input in order to be of benefit. These 'technique tips', as it were, need to be learnt. They may well surface naturally through a long process of trial and error - but that has already been done by somebody else, so we do not need to reinvent the wheel. As far as the bench press is concerned there are three techniques, I suggest, that are almost guaranteed to improve your performance.

The first concerns the width of grip used on the Olympic bar. I have already mentioned that the wider the grip the more stress is applied to the pectoral muscles as opposed to the triceps. A narrow grip on the other hand will put more stress on the triceps. Some professional weight lifters, having massive pectoral muscles, use a very wide grip which means the bar has less distance to travel to lockout position, possibly giving them a slight advantage. However, for the average person, the best technique is to use a grip of such a width so that when the bar is lowered to the chest the forearms are exactly perpendicular - not leaning out as in a wide grip, or leaning in as they would be in a very narrow grip.

In order to establish your own optimum grip get someone to watch when you lower the empty bar to your chest. While in that position slide your hands in or out as directed until the person checking you confirms your forearms are perpendicular. At that point look at the bar and note exactly where your hands are in relation to the small ring mark on the bar. These small ring marks are usually cut into the knurling at each side of the bar. In my particular case I know that if I place my middle finger exactly over the ring the width of my grip will be perfect. A smaller person may find they need to place their little finger over the ring mark - or even one inch inside it - to achieve their perfect grip. Just do the above experiment to find your own perfect grip, then remember it in relation to the mark, and then always stick to it.

A second technique which can help your performance is to consciously bring your shoulder blades together just before lifting the bar off the pins, and then to keep them together while pressing the bar up. This will have the effect of arching your back a little and raising your chest, thereby reducing the distance the bar has to descend. It sounds simple but it will take a few tries before this action becomes automatic.

Lastly, and again a technique that it is easy to forget to apply in practice, is to try and push with your feet as you press the bar up. Of course this is impossible since your legs are bent at roughly 90 degrees. However, by imagining you are standing up, and consciously trying to push up from your feet, you will ensure your whole body becomes involved in the lift and that your feet remain firmly planted on the floor.

Even if you forget to apply this technique, always keep your feet firmly on the floor to ensure stability with heavy weights. It is extremely bad form, and bad on safety grounds, to raise the legs and bend the knees up towards the chest - as unfortunately you will see many people doing.

This chapter on safe lifting, correct form and technique covers the last of the seven elements that I set out in Chapter 21 as being the essential ingredients of my optimal routine.
It may be worth repeating them here:

Warming Up
Overload
Sets and Repetitions
Balanced Training
Recovery
Nutrition
Safe Lifting, Correct Form & Technique.

While they are all important to any routine that aims to increase muscle mass in the most dramatic and efficient way, without overload there will certainly not be any dramatic increase in LBM, and quite probably no increase at all.

It is of course from increased muscle mass that all the other benefits will flow. I hope these 7 chapters have demonstrated just how straight forward, and enjoyable, gaining strength can be. It does not have to be time consuming - just 2 visits a week to the gym in order to reap all the benefits - and roll back your biological age by up to 20 years.

Chapter 29

The Downside

I have sometimes wondered if there is any downside. The only *possible* downside to strength training that I have ever experienced is that of having to upgrade part of my wardrobe. However, to me, the necessity of spending money on new shirts because of my increased chest size is happily accommodated. This is why I say that this is the only *possible* downside, because to many people buying new shirts is a positive upside - good retail therapy and truly earned.

I have come across a myth that larger muscles can slow you down in sports requiring quick reactions, such as tennis. I am not aware of any scientific tests that have been made to establish whether there is any relationship between muscle mass and reaction speed. As we have already seen, top tennis stars are now obliged to spend time in the weight room in order to maintain their game at the highest level. Over many years of increasing my strength on a measured basis I have not experienced one single negative side effect. ***Nor can I conceive of one.***

There are of course many downsides you are guaranteed to experience if you do ***nothing*** to develop your strength as you age – best illustrated I think by a few random facts:

- An average man has 35 percent less testosterone at 70 than he had at 30.
- About a quarter of all men are impotent by 70
- Between the ages of 40 and 70 a man loses 15 percent of his bone mass
- During the same period muscle mass will decrease and body fat increase, by approximately 20% respectively.

Pretty alarming statistics - but ***every*** single one of the above conditions is reversible by strength training. Building muscle is entirely under your control. You can transform your life right now. ***All*** of the 18 benefits that I have experienced are available to anyone, at any age. However, as I grow older I am most immediately impressed by my increasing strength and continuing ability to undertake absolutely any task that I choose. My chronological age has simply ceased to be an issue.

I set out to be my own guinea pig – and have become the living proof as to what an average person can achieve in a totally practical manner. The next chapter describes how you can monitor my progress and also receive ongoing help and support through my website.

Chapter 30

The Living Proof

The 18 benefits of strength training that I have identified have bettered my health in an incredible, but also in an everyday, practical way - and rolled back my biological age, I believe, by decades. As I write these words I know that when I go to the gym tomorrow I will be able to bench pres my bodyweight with something to spare. How much stronger can I get? What is my limit, and is getting even stronger going to benefit me further? Will the ever increasing weight finally have a detrimental effect on my joints, particularly on my shoulders?

Not being a professional bodybuilder, or weightlifter, I now no longer have the incentive to get stronger, other than to satisfy my curiosity - and to justify this book by being able to continue bench pressing my own bodyweight at the drop of a hat! I believe that so long as I just maintain my current level of strength I will continue to receive all of the benefits of a strong body by, of course, using it, and not losing it!

While that is all I need to do now to ensure continued mobility and thus independence right into advanced old age, curiosity will probably win out. That 1 rep max can probably be taken up a few notches over the next decade. After all, my biological age is now somewhere in the mid forties.

My website www.williamfaro.com will continue to monitor my progress into my seventies and eighties, and beyond, hopefully! More importantly it will also offer readers every help, support and encouragement. I hope you will visit it, even if only to satisfy your own curiosity. The 'links' button on the homepage will take you to the 'links & resources' page which will be continuously updated to direct you to what I believe to be the best illustrated exercises, and most useful associated articles and health news. By keeping the website constantly under review the problem of outdated links, references and addresses can be avoided. Questions and feedback can be submitted easily via the form (just click the 'contact us' button).

Those approaching retirement age and reading these words will almost certainly have a very strong desire to improve their health in any way that practically guarantees them many more active years on this planet. However, for anyone, at any stage of life, it is never too late, or too early, to start. Whatever your age I beg you to start living in your body - instead of dying in it. It truly is your only interface with reality.

To me the thought of growing physically weak as I age is no longer an option. To simply maintain my current strength now requires the minimum of effort. It just requires that I go on doing what I am doing. I recently heard about a Japanese gentleman who skis the Vallée Blanche at Chamonix every year. Nothing extraordinary about that, except that he is over 100 years old. As he explained, he has skied all his life and just forgot to stop. That, I believe, is all it takes to maintain a level of strength that will ensure all the benefits discussed in this book - just don't stop exercising.

At the risk of being repetitive I cannot stress enough that measured strength training, as covered in this book, will not turn you into a freak strongman. What it will do is ensure your independence right into advanced old age by sustaining and nurturing the natural strength that is your birthright.

Life is short enough, but the last third can be the best of all provided you maintain your health. With good health there are just so many pleasures that can be enjoyed for ever. Lose your health and you will almost certainly lose your mobility, independence and dignity as well. Strength training will ensure that never happens to you - and the best news is that it really is never too late to start.

THE END

Printed in the United Kingdom by
Lightning Source UK Ltd., Milton Keynes
142122UK00001B/61/A

9 781905 006748